How to
Stay Young
&Live Longer

The Definitive Guide to Anti-Aging

God Bless
Dr Marti Carda...

4/5/2012

by **Michael Lam,** MD, MPH, ABAAM
Maria Sulindro, MD, ABAAM
with **Dorine Tan,** RD, MS, MPH, ABBAHP

This is a work of non-fiction. The information, advices, and recommendations contained in this book are based on the training, personal experiences, opinions, and research of the authors. The information contained here is not intended to diagnose or treat any disease. They are intended for general information only and not as a substitute for consulting with your physician or other qualified health care provider. The publisher and the authors are not responsible for any adverse effects or consequences resulting from the use of any of the advice or recommendations in this book.

Published by Academy of Anti-Aging Research
1017 South Fair Oaks Avenue
Pasadena, CA 91105, USA
www.a3r.org

Printed in the United States of America
Reprinted in Singapore 1999, 2000, 2001.

Third Edition 2002
Designed and produced by FSTOP Pte Ltd
Cover Photo by FSTOP Pte Ltd

ISBN   0-9713036-0-6

Library of Congress Cataloging-in-Publication data

ABOUT THE AUTHORS

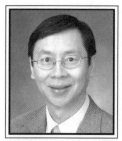

Michael Lam, MD, MPH, ABAAM, CNC is a specialist in Nutritional and Anti-Aging Medicine. He is currently the Director of Medical Education at the Academy of Anti-Aging Research, USA, overseeing the global education program for physicians and researchers in this field. Dr Lam received his Bachelor of Science degree from Oregon State University and his Doctor of Medicine degree from Loma Linda University School of Medicine, California. He also holds a Masters of Public Health degree in Preventive Health, and is Board Certified by the American Board of Anti-aging Medicine. Dr Lam is credited for being the first to formulate the three clinical phases of aging, and is a pioneer in using non-toxic natural compounds to treat age related degenerative diseases. His clinical specialty focuses on the use of optimum blends of nutritional supplementation that manipulates food, vitamins, natural hormones, herbs, enzymes, and mineral into specific protocols to rejuvenate cellular function. He is a recognized expert in nutritional medicine, being a Certified Nutritional Consultant and a Diplomat of the American Association of Nutritional Consultants. Dr Lam has been published extensively in this field. He has written over 50 scientific articles in natural medicine and the book *The Five Proven Secrets to Longevity*. He is listed in the International Who's Who of Professionals, serves as editor of the Journal of Anti-aging Research, and is a Board Examiner for the American Academy of Anti-aging Medicine.

To learn more about nutritional and anti-aging medicine, visit Dr Lam's commercial free and public education website

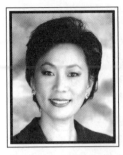 **Maria Sulindro, MD, ABAAM** has been actively practicing Anti-Aging Medicine for over a decade and is the Medical Director of the Anti-Aging Center in Pasadena, California. She completed her Physical Medicine and Rehabilitation residency program at the University of California at Los Angeles in 1987. Her anti-aging program is world-renowned. She is Board Certified by the American Board of Anti-Aging Medicine and is a diplomat of the American College for the Advancement of Medicine. Dr Sulindro is the co-author of The Five Proven Secrets to Longevity. She is also the founder and President of the Academy of Anti-Aging Research, a professional organization offering Fellowship Programs with certified continuing medical education awards to health professionals around the world (further information is available at www. *MariaMD.com*

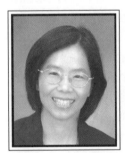 **Dorine Tan, RD, MS, MPH, ABAAHP** is a Registered Clinical Dietician, specializing in the research and development of dietary protocol in an anti-aging setting. She received her bachelor's degree in Dietetics and Nutrition, a Masters of Science in Nutrition, and a Masters of Public Health from Loma Linda University, California. Ms Tan is also Board Certified by the American Board of Anti-Aging Health Practitioners.

CONTENTS

CHAPTER **FIVE**

HOW TO GET THE MOST OUT OF THIS BOOK

To help you learn about anti-aging, we have **highlighted** some special tips and information throughout the book that you need to know for optimum anti-aging health.

There are also boxes that appear throughout each of the chapters. The boxes below appear in the chapters of this book and their purposes are as stated.

HOW TO ADD 20 YEARS TO YOUR LIFE ...
By simply following these tips, you can add years to your life and increase the quality of life as well.

ANTI-AGING TOP TENS
This is a list of the top tens related to anti-aging, including the Top Ten Anti-Aging Supplements, Do's, Don'ts, Motivation Tips, Foods, etc.

ACTION PRINCIPLE
These are short motivational pieces that you can remember to help you stay on track in your anti-aging program. Remember, anti-aging is a lifestyle change, and having the right mental attitude is the key to success.

FREQUENTLY ASKED ANTI-AGING QUESTIONS
The answers to your most frequently asked anti-aging questions.

FOREWORD

Only a century ago, the average life expectancy was 42 years. Today, it has almost doubled. This is due not only to advances in medicine and technology but, more importantly, to proper nutrition and lifestyle adjustments. The definition of aging as a natural and irreversible course of events has passed. Today, we see healthy and active seniors well into their 90s. There are over 70,000 centenarians in United States alone and this number is expected to double in the next five to ten years. In fact, those over 85 years old represent the fastest growing segment of the population in the world.

Anti-aging as a medical specialty has evolved only in the last 20 years with advancements in medical research and technology. Aging is certainly not inevitable if you know what to do.

Patients from around the globe seek anti-aging specialists for one reason only – **HOW TO STAY YOUNG AND LIVE LONGER.** They know about wellness, they know about exercise, and they know about nutritional supplementation. They consult specialists because they want the best and the latest information on how they can maintain their youth and prolong their lives. They know that the best-kept secrets in any field are often not readily available. They know that from research to clinical studies to mass public acceptance is a process that often takes from 20 to 30 years. These people do not want to wait. They want to know what to do and they want it immediately.

They want to know:
a. Steps to make them younger today — the exact nutrients, the exact hormone and the exact dosage.

b. How to reverse the **sub-clinical** state of disease that many "normal" adults already have (but may not be symptomatic), such as failing memory, high blood pressure, high blood sugar and heart disease.
c. How to naturally prevent or reverse **active disease states** they already have, such as stroke and cancer.

These patients are the best teachers for anti-aging physicians. Anti-aging concepts are new and non-traditional. They challenge us and force us to do our research. In other words, they propel us to higher grounds of excellence.

This book has come about in response to many requests to have a simple summary of the salient points of anti-aging medicine. This book contains many excerpts from the bigger volume, *The Five Proven Secrets to Longevity*, by Drs Michael Lam and Maria Sulindro.

The following five pillars of anti-aging will be discussed in turn.
1. Optimal Anti-Aging Supplementation
2. Natural Hormone Enhancement
3. Anti-Aging Specific Exercises
4. Anti-Aging Nutrition
5. Stress Reduction

The book will end with a summary of over 100 key anti-aging strategies you can start using today and objective tools to measure your success going forward.

Welcome to the ageless society!

Clayton Varga, MD, MHSM
Dean, Academy of Anti-Aging Research

MESSAGE FROM DR MICHAEL LAM

I t was not too long ago when our exploration of the human body was limited to the organs and their gross pathology. Today, we are able to travel to the inner sanctuary of the cell, well into the amino acid structure of the DNA. The rapid speed of such discovery means that **many of our traditional understanding of health issues need constant revising and updating.**

The concept of aging is one such issue. Research has shown that our life expectancy is not pre-destined and something can be done to change it. Those of us who have dedicated our lives to anti-aging medicine believe that **aging should be viewed more appropriately as a collection of chronic degenerative diseases**, such as arthritis, diabetes and loss of memory. The good news is that the majority of these conditions can be reversed and cured in this early stage by natural and non -toxic compounds that have been around for centuries but ignored by the medical community in the past 150 years.

The anti-aging information presented in this book is time-tested and real. It does not work 100% of the time because genes determine 30% of one's longevity. However, one can modulate the other 70%.

In the end, we strive to strike a difference between your chronological and physical age. We want you to be physically younger than what you are chronologically. Those that follow our anti-aging program have seen a difference of 10 years or more easily and this age difference increases as you age. It is not uncommon for a patient to have a physical age up to 20 years younger than their chronological age when they hit their 80's. In other words, they may have a body of a 60-year-old when they are in their 80's.

The practice of Nutritional and Anti-Aging Medicine is not just about living longer. It is about the opportunity to live a full and happy life. When you follow our anti-aging program, you are giving yourself and your loved ones the ultimate gift – the gift of time.

Michael Lam, MD, MPH, ABAAM,CNC
Nutritional and Anti-Aging Medicine Specialist,
Board Certified, American Board of Anti-Aging Medicine

CHAPTER ONE

INTRODUCTION TO AGING

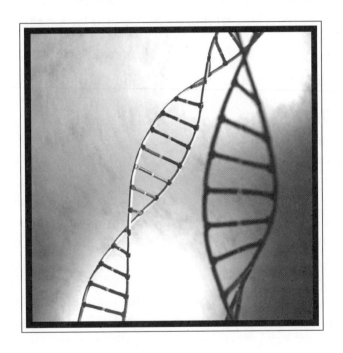

"Youth has no age."

Pablo Picasso

Health experts say that the average person spends the last 12 years of life depending on others for his daily living needs. It is never too late to increase your chances of enjoying a healthier and longer life.

Do you know how to prevent, deter and even reverse aging diseases and conditions?

Would you like to look and feel young again, rarely get sick and live a lifestyle with more energy and less pain than ever before?

Only a generation ago, terms like free radicals, oxidative stress and mitochondrial disease were words used in research laboratories. Today, these are household words. Only a generation ago, it was unthought of to link infections with gastric ulcers. Today, it is a proven fact. When AIDS first surfaced, many believed it was a curse from God. Yet, our thinking has changed, because science compels us to. The explosion of scientific research on aging is truly frightening. As we know today, aging is not "natural" at all. In fact, it is nothing more than a collection of common aging conditions and diseases such as high blood pressure, cancer, heart disease and diabetes. The human body is traumatized on a daily basis if one is exposed to an unhealthy diet, environmental pollution, and stressful lifestyle. Researchers report that 90% of all adult illnesses and conditions are due to the degenerative processes associated with aging.

These diseases are common in old age. If you could be young again, you would not have to worry as much about these diseases.

TOP 10 SYMPTOMS OF AGING

1. **Stained Teeth** – too much coffee or cigarettes.
2. **Cracks in corner of mouth** – Vitamin B deficiencies.
3. **Bleeding gums and periodontal disease** – take Vitamin C, CoQ10, and bioflavinoids.
4. **Dry and flaky hair** – take B vitamins and essential fatty acids.
5. **Skin bruising** – take Vitamin C, K, and bioflavinoids.
6. **Nails splitting and cracking** – take calcium, zinc, protein, and fatty acids.
7. **Irregular heart beat** – avoid caffeine; take magnesium and CoQ10.
8. **Pale tongue** – represents anemia.
9. **Constipation** – take fiber, digestive enzymes.
10. **Memory loss** – take gingko, phospatidylserine.

PHASES OF AGING

Anti-aging medicine and research now defines aging as nothing more than a disease state characterized by three phases:

1. Sub-Clinical Phase, ages 25 to 35

Most hormone levels start to decrease. Growth hormone level, for example, has already fallen by approximately 14% by age 35. Environmental pollution, poor diet and stress cause free radical formation and cellular damage that is not visible to the naked eye. Outwardly, there are few clinical symptoms. While you may look and feel good, internal cellular damage is already happening. Like cancer, in its early stages of development, there are no signs and symptoms detectable by conventional standards. You look and feel "normal", but in reality you are in the sub-clinical phase of this disease, whether you like it or not.

2. Transition Phase, ages 35 to 45

By age 45, production of many hormones has fallen by more than 25% and biomarkers are beginning to show significant signs of aging. Clinical symptoms such as decreased visual acuity, graying of hair, increased pigmentation of the skin and decreased strength and energy are making their presence felt on the outside. Internally, cellular damage by free radical continues, where the rate of damage depends on your lifestyle. If not controlled or slowed down, mutational changes within the cell may lead to cancer.

3. Clinical Phase, ages 45 and above

Most hormone production continues to decline, including DHEA, melatonin, growth hormone and male and female sexual hormones. The rate of decline accelerates as we get older until age 70 or thereabouts. Outwardly, early signs and symptoms of aging seen during the transition phase worsen. The skin is further dehydrated and thinned as collagen fibers break down. We call these irreversible lines "wrinkles." Musculo-skeletal joints degeneration become painfully obvious as arthritis sets in. Fatigue and loss of energy follow us everywhere. Chronic illnesses such as hypertension and diabetes become more apparent as organs begin to fail. Internally, our cells succumb to assaults.

Atherosclerosis and cancer becomes the leading cause of death and disability.

HOW TO ADD 20 YEARS TO YOUR LIFE ...

Drive a heavy car and wear a seat belt – Add 0.6 years.

Studies have shown that driving a car weighing more than 3,500 pounds increases your chances of surviving a car crash by ten times.

UNDERSTANDING THE ANTI-AGING PHYSICIAN

As we can see, the aging process really starts in the early 20s. Many degenerative diseases commonly associated with aging (eg. thinning of the skin, decrease in muscle strength) takes an average of 20 years or more to develop to become symptomatic or visible.

The fallacy that the absence of outright detectable symptoms of aging and the failure of confirmation by current laboratory tests equate to a "normal" body must be dispelled. What is "normal" by traditional medial standards should not be so considered from an anti-aging perspective. Most of the current tests are not sensitive enough to detect cellular changes occurring within the body. Many people who are "normal" may already be in the sub-clinical phase of degenerative diseases, such as hypertension, osteoarthritis, atherosclerosis and diabetes.

In order to truly practice anti-aging medicine, the anti-aging physicians, therefore, must re-define common laboratory

reference standards into two groups: standards for those who are clinically sick with active diseases and for those who are considered "normal" but actually in sub-clinical phases of degenerative diseases characteristic of the aging process.

For example, a fasting blood sugar of 100-120 mg/dl is sub-optimum and reflects the sub-clinical or "pre-diabetic" phase. Yet, few know how to reverse this pre-diabetic phase other than through dietary control and exercise. The knowledgeable anti-aging physician recognizes that the ideal fasting blood sugar should be close to 90 mg/dl and treatments using natural and non-toxic alternatives to reach this state are administered. Drugs will only be used when needed. The body is not a light switch, but is a miraculous machine that often gives advance signals to warn us of impending diseases.

Aging is not inevitable once the concept of undetectable sub-clinical disease states are understood. Those who are pro-active and treat aging as a disease can deter the aging process. Since the aging process begins in the cell, **anti-aging physicians set down a treatment** strategy to maximize the life span of each cell in the body. When the cell lives longer, you will live longer, too.

The understanding of cellular function is, therefore, of paramount importance to any anti-aging specialist and those who are interested to live longer. Knowing the cause of cellular damage will lead us to the discovery of treatment, either in the form of drugs or natural alternative means to help the cell defend and renew itself. The science of ortho-molecular medicine is dedicated to such a cause. It is the discipline of nutritional therapy that advocates the use of a whole food diet and nutritional supplementation to produce a state of optimum health.

Anti-aging medicine incorporates many of the principals of ortho-molecular medicine to retard aging and rejuvenate the body in addition to the following disciplines: nutrition, biochemistry, cell biology, physiology, general medicine, immunology, allergy, endocrinology, pharmacology, toxicology, neurology, gastroenterology, nephrology and physical medicine.

The following therapeutic modalities fall into the realm of the anti-aging physician: hormonal replacement therapy, vitamins, minerals, amino acids, essential fatty acids, fibers, enzymes, antibodies, antigens, cell therapy, chelation therapy, hydrotherapy, thermal therapy, detoxification, exercise, biofeedback, psychotherapy and others. Drugs and medicines are used in conjunction with non-invasive natural and the least toxic modality to achieve optimum health.

THE SECRET IS IN THE DETAILS

Knowing what to do in detail in each of the modalities is the key to anti-aging. Even if you believe that the nutritional approach is a correct one, you may not know the dosage, the frequency and the contraindications, if any, of each nutrient. Research had shown that the average consumer who is knowledgeable on nutrition actually knows more than the average physician. This may be startling to you but the fact is that the average doctor receives less than ten hours of nutritional training in four years of medical school curriculum. This is indeed frightening, but real. In fact, **doctors' and hospitals' errors are the third leading cause of death in America according to a recent article published by the most widely circulated medical periodical in the world, the *Journal of the American Medical Association*. The average doctor's life expectancy is no longer that of the**

average person. Yet, these are professionals who are supposed to be armed with the latest knowledge on how to extend life. The current generation of doctors are trained and focused on treating degenerative diseases when they are clinically active, but not on treating diseases when they are in the sub-clinical phase characteristic of the aging process.

For example, anti-aging research has now proven that optimum levels of anti-aging nutritional supplementation is one important tool to deter and slow the aging process. The question is: what intake is optimum? What intake is too much? And what intake is too little?

No matter what nutritional supplements you are taking, ensure that they include the following.

1. A precise blend of antioxidant-rich ingredients that fight free radicals, gives you strong anti-aging protection,significantly boosts your immunity and nourishes all the life-sustaining cells in your body.
2. A strong, well-balanced nutritional cocktail to keep your heart healthy and pumping strongly, increase your immunity, maintain the proper acid/base balance and help clear clogged vessels of unwanted plaques.
3. A powerful energy-boosting complex that gives you long-lasting stamina and endurance.
4. Strong nutrients to balance your blood sugar and control insulin secretion.

Anti-aging research now also tells us that hormone deficiencies are key factors in accelerating pre-mature aging. There are various hormones in our body, the most important of which is the growth hormone.

Nearly all individuals over the age of 25 have deficiency in Human Growth Hormone. Your body generally reaches its peak performance around age 25, which is when the **growth hormone is at its highest level**. From that point onwards, the growth hormone level in the body declines steadily and the natural progression of aging starts taking its toll on the body. Those interested in anti-aging should consider some form of **Growth Hormone rejuvenator (also called a secretagogue)**. This is a nutritional supplementation that is derived from natural food sources. Human Growth Hormone level in the body declines with age at a rate of approximately 14% every decade from the peak. Growth Hormone reaches far beyond the scope of many hormones. Its effect not only prevents biological aging but also significantly reverses many age-related signs and symptoms. Numerous beneficial effects with the increase of growth hormone level were reported, such as the reduction of pain, loss of fat, reduction of wrinkles, growth of hair, better sleep, increase in muscle tone, improvements in sex drive, brain function, vision, immune function and cholesterol profile.

As you age, the Growth Hormone is stored in the pituitary gland in your body, but is not being released in adequate amounts. The proper secretogogue (including those made from peptides, amino acids or a combination) acts on the pituitary, causing it to release growth hormone in proper amounts. Choosing the right secretagogue is the key.

In addition to optimal anti-aging supplementation and natural hormonal enhancement using secretagogues, a special anti-aging diet, precision anti-aging exercises and stress management should be included in a comprehensive anti-aging program.

We will examine each of these topics in more detail in the following chapters.

TOP 10 FACTS ABOUT AGING

1. **Every 7.7 seconds**, one American turns 50 years old.
2. There are **70 million baby boomers** in the US alone.
3. **Cancer** is the number one cause of death, followed by heart disease and stroke.
4. There are **70,000 centenarians** at 1996. This is projected to be 160,000 by year 2010.
5. **Cancer** – one out of two men and one out of three women will experience some form of cancer in their lifetime. The chance of developing invasive cancer by age 60 is 1 in 12 for men and 1 in 12 for women. By age 79, the chances for developing invasive cancer increase to one in three in men and one in five in women.
6. Many baby boomers are **expected to live to 100** years in an active lifestyle.
7. 80% of baby boomers **do not eat a balanced diet**, and only 33% exercise regularly.
8. **Aging is a treatable disease** that is 70% related to lifestyle and only 30% related to genetics.
9. **80 million** have elevated cholesterol, 60 million have high blood pressure, 41 million have arthritis and 16 million have diabetes in the US.
10. More visits are made to **alternative health care providers** than to conventional medical doctors in the US.

CHAPTER TWO

WHEN YOU'RE 45 …

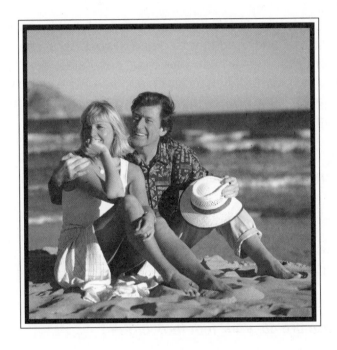

*"The man who views the world
at 50 the same as he did at 20 has
wasted 30 years of his life."*
Muhammad Ali

There are many myths about aging, with stories ranging from reduced brain capacity to decreased libido. Many of these myths are just that, myths that have no scientific basis. The following is a list of the most common aging myths and the truth about them.

ENERGY
When you are 45, you do not have the energy you had when you were 30.

False. Low energy levels are more often related to poor aerobic fitness, stress and inadequate sleep. Those who are in shape have plenty of energy well into their seventies. A proper diet, exercise, supplementation program and adequate sleep will boost your energy level tremendously. They will make up for the physiological decline that comes naturally with age.

SMELL
Your sense of smell declines as you grow older.

True. Between the ages of 40 and 60, your sense of smell declines by 10% to as much as 50%. To keep your sense of smell functioning properly, expose them to various fragrances a few times a day. Stimulating your sense of smell can slow down the loss.

FEET
When you are 45, your feet look bigger.

True. Your feet continue to grow in both length and width throughout your life by up to one full shoe size between ages 20 and 50 due to softening of the bones and stretching of the ligaments of the foot. This is normal.

TASTE
When you are 45, food does not tastes as good.

True. Your sense of smell controls about 90% of your sense of taste, so food tastes more bland as you get older as your sense of smell gradually deteriorates. As a result, you will crave for more sweet and saltier foods. To combat "bland" tasting food, you should chew your food more. This allows more aroma to reach your nose. Chewing your food longer also allows more digestive enzymes to go to work, which in turn facilitates digestion.

HEALING
When you are 45, cuts and injuries do not heal as quickly.

True. The rate of healing may decrease because of age-related reduction in blood flow that slow the healing response. You should keep antibiotic ointment and hydrogen peroxide handy for cuts. These keep out germs and hastens the healing process.

HOW TO ADD 20 YEARS TO YOUR LIFE ...

Prevent Stroke – Add 3 years

Strokes are caused by clogged vessels in the brain. People who have strokes become debilitated and even if they recover, they are usually never the same as before.
- Keep arteries unclogged and blood pressure down through proper diet, weight control, exercise and stress reduction.
- Keep blood vessels strong and flexible with antioxidants, vitamin C, L-Proline, L-Lysine and ascobyl palmitate.
- Keep homocycteine and lipoprotein (a) (key independent factors of heart disease) level low by adding folic acid, vitamin C, B12 and B6 to a daily supplement program.

SEX
When you are 45, great sex is hard to come by.

False. Great sex has both a psychological as well as physical component. You may not have two to three climaxes a night, but that is because you have gotten better at having just one. The quantity may have decreased, but the quality has probably increased. Most people in optimum health are able to have great sex well into their 70s.

SLEEP
When you are 45, you do not sleep as soundly.

True. Brief moments of spontaneous awakening (which is a normal part of the sleep cycle) increase with age. Most aging adults find it necessary to wake up in the middle of the night because of a need to urinate. For better sleep, stick to a regular sleep schedule and avoid caffeine and heavy meals just before bed. Make sure you sleep in a totally dark room in order to maximize melatonin production by your body.

SWEAT
When you are 45, you sweat more easily.

True. As you age, your body cools itself less efficiently, so you could be operating at a higher temperature during a workout. Therefore, your body has to sweat more to keep cool. This is normal. Sweating is also an excellent way of detoxification.

URINATION
When you are 45, you cannot hit the urinal from three paces anymore.

True. Beginning at age 25, hormonal changes may cause your prostate to enlarge gradually and symptoms such as frequent urination often surfaces after age 40. All men above age 40 should regularly check for prostate cancer. Also, men should consider taking Saw Palmetto, nettle roots and pygeum on a prophylactic basis after age 35 for optimal prostate health.

TOP 10 ANTI-AGING DON'TS

1. **Don't** rely on food alone for all your nutritional needs.
2. **Don't** let free radicals run wild in your body.
3. **Don't** think that medical prescription drugs are your only answer.
4. **Don't** neglect powerful phytonutrients.
5. **Don't** eat white bread or junk food.
6. **Don't** eat the same food everyday.
7. **Don't** lead a sedentary lifestyle.
8. **Don't** be negative in your attitude towards life.
9. **Don't** procrastinate in seeing a doctor.
10. **Don't** let life pass you by.

HAIR ON CALVES
When you are 45, your calves start going bald.

True. It is very common for your calves to start going bald, especially from the sock line down. The reason is that less blood moves through the lower extremities, and with this lower oxygen delivery, hair follicles gradually atrophy and die.

PENIS SIZE
When you are 45, your penis is smaller.

False. It may look smaller if the rest of you is getting bigger. When you gain weight, the fat pad on the pubic bone around the base of your penis becomes thicker and that can hide up to an inch of the length of your penis.

FAT BURNING
When you are 45, your body cannot burn fat as fast as it did when you were 25.

False. While your metabolism does slow down somewhat, the more likely explanation for any weight gain is a change in habits (eating the same amount of food and exercising less). Simply exercise more and eat less.

MEMORY
When you are 45, your memory goes.

FREQUENT ANTI-AGING QUESTION

Q: Does sexual activity help you to live longer?

Many studies have been conducted in this area in the past few decades. Most of them confirmed that an active sex life does increase longevity. The difference can be as much as five to ten years. Energetic sex, the researchers say, can help reduce fatty tissues and also release endorphins that combat anxiety, stress and other negative emotions. Studies have found that such negative feelings increased a person's risk for chronic illness, including heart disease. Other researchers have found that a healthy sex life is linked to a stronger immune system, fewer bouts of sickness, and overall better mental health. Regular sexual activity is an important part of life.

False. Our memory does not deteriorate significantly until we hit age 70. Most likely, there is information overload and you cannot remember all the things you wanted. Morning is the best time for concentration and avoiding distractions if you are looking to get things done. Keep your mind active but not overloaded.

HEARING
When you are 45, your hearing goes down.

False. Most likely, the hearing problems have more to do with all the noises you have been exposed to (motorcycles, lawn mowers, etc.) causing hearing loss, instead of your age.

MENTAL DEXTERITY
When you are 45, it takes you longer to figure things out.

False. Your mental function is like a muscle. To get maximum performance, you have to use it. Start by learning something challenging, like a musical instrument, reading or painting. Nutrients such as phosphatidylserine and gingko biloba can also help keep brain cells healthy and functioning at their optimum state.

EARLOBES
When you are 45, your earlobes look bigger.

True. Earlobes lengthen at the rate of 0.22 mm per year after adulthood. At age 50, it is 0.25 inches longer, compared to what they were at age 30.

TOILET TIME
When you are 45, you spend more time in the toilet.

True. As you get older, the contractions in your colon and rectum are not as well coordinated. Therefore, you may be more constipated. Include vegetables, fibres, bran cereal, digestive enzymes and sufficient water in your diet. This is a good way to increase regularity and decrease your toilet time.

HEARTBURN
When you are 45, you get heartburn more often.

True. The valve that keeps stomach acid out of your esophagus starts to lose its factory-tight seal and gastric reflux occurs. To minimize the effects of acid reflux, do not sleep until at least two hours after eating.

ACTION PRINCIPLE

Be Honest With Yourself

The first rule of war is: know yourself. In order to know yourself, you must first acknowledge and then compensate for your weaknesses. Ask your friends and mentors: What am I good at? In what areas should I improve? What do you do better than most people? Do not be afraid to ask for advice or help and do not be afraid to listen to the answers. Reflect and learn. Knowing yourself allows you to plan your days for peak performance.

Accept your limitations. Accept your circumstances. Be the best you can be internally, and your beauty and confidence will be reflected externally.

Sometimes, we may not like what we see. The fact is that the truth hurts, sometimes. Do not get discouraged. Congratulate yourself for being honest, as it is the first step to wisdom.

CHAPTER **THREE**

CASE STUDIES

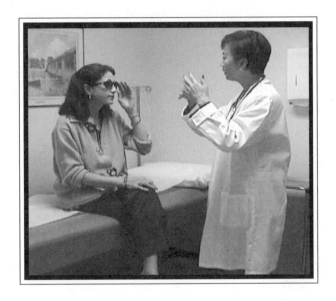

*"I don't want to get to the end of my life
and find that I have just lived the length of it.
I want to have lived the width of it as well."*

Diane Ackerman

The joy of seeing our patients cured from degenerative diseases such as hypertension, cancer, diabetes, cardiac arrhythmia, high cholesterol and hormonal imbalance and return to a youthful state is indeed rewarding. For the first time in medical history, we are truly able to be real physicians, actually reversing and curing many age-related degenerative diseases instead of treating symptoms of these diseases. This is what makes anti-aging as a medical specialty so exciting.

Here are some real life case histories of patients we have treated. While they come to see us from across the globe and represent a cross-segment of the population, they have one wish in common: to cure their diseases naturally instead of simply suppressing symptoms through traditional medical protocols involving prescription drugs.

Their successes are a testament of the effectiveness of anti-aging and nutritional medicine. The identities of the patients have been concealed for privacy reasons.

ANTI-AGING CASE HISTORY

This is a typical case study of a well-executed and comprehensive anti-aging program.

John is a **61-year-old** successful businessman. He is 5 feet 3 inches tall and weighs 135 pounds.

John's main **complaints are: mild joint pain, back pain, lack of energy, lack of libido, hair loss, worsening visual acuity, loss of short-term memory, thinning skin, and age spots.**

His has no prior surgeries or allergies, and is currently not on medication. He has been thoroughly evaluated by other physicians for his complaint, including extensive testing. **He was told that his complaints are "normal for his age", and there is nothing more that can be done to rid his concerns**. He has a family history of diabetes, hypertension, and stroke.

On this initial visit, an extensive history form was completed with a complete review of systems. In addition to review by the physician, the data is fed into a computer for analysis and calculation of physical age versus chronological age. **His chronological age is 61, and physical age shows 63. He is actually older than he is.** His physical examination is essentially normal for his age.

In addition to traditional laboratory studies such as chemistry panel, complete blood count, complete urine analysis, the following **anti-aging baseline studies were done:**

1. **Hormonal panel** including free testosterone, total testosterone, DHEA, and SHBG.
2. **Cancer marker** studies including PSA.
3. **Cardiac panel** including homocysteine, ferritin, C Reactive Protein, Lipoprotein (a).
4. **Red pack cell studies of minerals,** including calcium, magnesium, potassium, copper, zinc, iron, manganese, chromium, selenium, boron, vanadium, and molybdenum.
5. **Red pack cell toxic element study** including Arsenic, Cadmium, Lead, and Mercury.
6. **24-hour urine toxic screen** (pre and post provocation test with DMPS).
7. **Bone density test**.
8. **Ultra-fast CT scan** (EBCT) of the heart and coronary blood vessel.

9. **Thyroid panel** including TIBC, TSH, Free T3, Free T4.
10. **Lipid panel** including total cholesterol, HDL cholesterol, LDL cholesterol, and triglyceride.

Anti-aging bio-maker studies include:

1. Arterial stiffness index.
2. Postural blood pressure readings.
3. Postural resting pulse.
4. Body analyzer study for fat, lean mass, water, weight.
5. Forced vital capacity.
6. Flexibility test.
7. Static balance test.

Result of Initial Studies are:

1. EBCT (Ultrafast CT Scan) test show calcification in the left anterior descending coronary artery consistent with **moderate plaque burden** (Calcium lesion of index of 4 and Ca score of 197).
2. Toxic element study showing **mercury toxicity** at 0.058 (normal 0.01) and borderline Lead toxicity at 0.087 (normal 0.09).
3. **Elevated arterial stiffness** index with score of 108 (normal under 70).
4. **Elevate body fat** of 25%. Goal is 20%.
5. **Low body water** of 56.8% (normal 60-65%).
6. **Elevated body weight** at 8% above normal for age.
7. **Elevated fasting glucose** of 133 (goal 90 mg/dl).
8. **Low IGF-1** of 150 mg/ml (normal above 200 for his age).
9. **Slightly below average level of free testosterone.**

Diagnosis

1. **Aging in Advanced Clinical Phase.** Post andropause.
2. **Systolic Hypertension.** BP 151/80 with moderate arterial stiffness.
3. **Adult growth hormone deficiency syndrome.**
4. **Moderate coronary occlusive disease** evidenced by ultrafast CT scan.
5. **Sub-clinical dehydration.**
6. **Adult onset diabetes mellitus (NIIDM Type 2).**
7. **Toxic metal overload** (mercury and lead).

Treatment Goals

1. Reverse coronary artery occlusive disease naturally by reducing plaque formation in the coronary artery by 40%.
2. Reverse systolic hypertension naturally to under 120 mg.
3. Increase arterial flexibility (reduce stiffness) to further reduce diastolic pressure naturally.
4. Reverse Diabetes and normalize blood sugar naturally to a fasting blood sugar of under 100 mg/dl.
5. Increase libido naturally to be consistent with age and to be able to perform sexual function at least three times a week.
6. Enhancement of endogenous hormonal system.
7. Detoxification of toxic metal from the body to desirable level.

Discussion

This is a 61-year-old patient (on no medication) who is **considered normal by traditional medical standards and blood test. He has generalized complaints consistent with advance stages of aging in its clinical phase,** toxic mercury and lead toxicity evidenced by pack red blood cell studies not detected by traditional laboratory test. He has had a compromised cardiovascular system evidenced by high coronary artery calcium, high blood pressure, and moderate arterial stiffness. In addition, many of his complaints can be related to adult growth hormone deficiency syndrome. He is well into the **clinical phase of aging,** and **proactive steps are needed to reverse the gradual decline in hormonal and physical function.** Steps are also needed to prevent further oxidative stress and free radical attacks on the cellular structure to deter the aging process and prevent cancer at his high-risk age.

Plan of Action

Patient was started on the following regiment.

1. **Optimum nutritional supplementation optimized for his age, sex, and physical condition.**
   - Anti-Aging high potency optimum nutritional supplementation program am and pm pack specific for male over the age of 45 years
   - Brain formula – one a day
   - Eye formula – one a day
   - Heart formula – two a day
   - Joint formula – two a day
   - DHEA 25 mg – two a day
   - Melatonin 1 mg – one a day
   - Pregnenolone – one a day
   - MSM – one a day
   - Ca/Magnesium – two a day
   - Probiotics – one a day
   - Ascorbic acid 1000 mg – one a day

Over 70 nutrients are packed in a nutritional cocktail designed to accomplish the following:
- Rebalance the microcirculation system.
- Reboost the immune system.
- Re-establish intestinal flora.
- Regulate internal ecology (pH and cell respiration).
- Repair damaged organ.
- Reduce oxidative stress to key organs.
- Replace deficient nutrients.
- Return blood sugar to normal level.

2. **Oral Chelation** program for metal toxicity:
   EDTA-Mg 300mg – 3 tablet 2 times a day.
3. **Hormonal enhancement:**
   MD Gee-h oral secretagogue – two in the evening.
4. **Colon Detoxification** through herbal tea.
5. **Triglyceride and blood pressure control** with soluble fiber:
   15 gram two to three times a day plus diet modification.
6. **Blood sugar control** with chromium polynicotinate supplementation to normalize blood sugar.
7. **Increase water** intake to ten glasses a day.
8. **Anti-aging exercise program.**
9. **Anti-aging diet program.**
10. **Anti-aging stress reduction program.**

Follow up interval and frequency

The patient was seen **every three months.** During these visits, modifications to his regiment of nutritional supplements were made.

Progress Report

1 . **After three months,** repeat ultra-fast CT scan of coronary vessels showed a **24% reduction in calcium plaque in** the left anterior descending coronary artery.

2. **After three months** on the program, red pack cell mineral analysis showed:
   - **3% increase in magnesium level**
   - blunted increase in chromium despite increased supplemental chromium intake. Suggested possible insulin resistant. Chromium level was still sub-optimal. Further adjustments were made to normalize sugar.
   - **10% increase in selenium level**
   - **60% reduction of mercury**
   - **60% reduction of lead**

3. **Arterial stiffness index reduced by 25% in three months** from 108 to 83. This signifies a younger and more elastic vascular system. This was further **reduced to 50% in one year** from 108 to 56.

4. **Systolic blood pressure reduced by 6% over three months** from 151 to 142 , and **13% over one year** from 151 to 132.

5. **Diastolic pressure reduced by 12 %** from already healthy level of 80 to 70 within 3 months and stabilized at around that level.

6. **Pulse reduced by 15%** from 71 to 62 beats per minute after three months and stabilized at that level.

7. His triglyceride level went up from 62 to 124 mg/dl over the course of a year. While this is still within normal limits, it reflects the patient's high intake of sugar in the diet and not following the anti-aging diet as closely as he should.

8. **IGF-1 (indicative of growth hormone) increased by 18%** from 150 to 178 mg/ml on oral secretagogue. Patient tried growth hormone injection but developed headache and it was abandoned after two weeks.

9. **Fasting Glucose reduced from 133 to 118 mg/dl within the first three months,** but later creeps back up to 136 when growth hormone **injection** was started. His sugar level stabilized once growth hormone injection was discontinued. Oral secretagogue did not affect the blood sugar level.

10. **Body fat reduced by 21%** in 12 months from 25% to 19.1%, reaching the goal of no more than 20%.
11. **Lean body mass increased by 10%** over 12 months from 75% to 80.9%, reaching the goal of 80%.
12 **Water composition increased by 10%** from 56.8% to 61%, reaching the goal of 60%.
13. Weight maintain at 8% above ideal body weight for age, but due to the body composition change, the body is in healthy state compared to moderately overweight before.

After one year on anti-aging program

1. Target organs have shown consistent improvement.
2. Glandular system rejuvenated at the rate of 10 years in 12 months.
3. Cardiovascular system rejuvenated at the rate of 10 years in 12 months.
4. Physical, fat and muscle index improved.
5. Diabetes still not fully reversed. More modulation is needed.
6. Physical age is now approximately 53, while chronological age is 61.

Conclusion

John is a typical patient who has embarked on and followed an anti-aging program successfully. His personalized anti-aging program addresses the five pillars of anti-aging medicine: anti-aging exercise, anti-aging diet, natural hormonal enhancement, stress reduction and optimum nutritional supplementation. Being a businessman on the go, his stress level did not reduce. After one year on the program, he is physically ten years younger. His blood pressure is better than most 30 years younger. His body composition has changed to reflect less fat and more protein. His blood sugar has stabilized, though not yet optimized. Physically, John has more energy. Mentally, he is more sharp. His libido has improved. His concentration and memory ability is better than before. **In John's own words:** *"I feel 10 years younger."* **What John now knows is that he feels that way because he *IS* physically and functionally ten years younger!**

CARDIAC ARRYTHMIA STABILIZED NATURALLY

ML was a physician referred to us by a cardiologist. He was a healthy 45-year-old male when he developed a fast and irregular heart rate called atrial fibrillation. At times, his heart rate would beat up to 120 times a minute and he had to go to the emergency room for help. ML also had a mitral valve prolapse, intermittent chest pain and a strong family history of diabetes. ML was very dedicated to his work. He maintained a full schedule and was a typical type A highly strung person.

As a physician, ML knew that the traditional medical protocol used by cardiologists to slow down and control heart rate was only a band-aid approach at best. He was on drugs for about three months and decided to stop to find natural and alternative methods to treat his condition.

ML started on our anti-aging program, using nutritional supplements to fortify his heart function. He was started on a strong regimen of antioxidants to prevent free radical damage to his mitochondria. Over the course of 12 months, a combination of anti-aging supplements and lifestyle adjustments were used to gradually wean him off his medication, while ensuring that his normal heart rhythm was maintained.

His irregular heart rate has not recurred. He was able to run a half marathon recently. His blood pressure is close to that of a 20-year-old. An ultra-fast CT scan of his coronary vessels has shown up clear. His heart is as strong as that of a man years younger. **This is what anti-aging medicine is all about: the ability to cure diseases that traditional western medicine has difficulty controlling.**

COLON CANCER IN REMISSION

MJ is a middle-aged legal secretary who comes from a family with a history of ovarian and colon cancer. She had her first colon cancer surgery in her mid-30s. By the time she came to see us, she had already had three surgeries, chemotherapy and radiotherapy. She had just completed the last course of radiotherapy and vowed never to go back. She was very frightened of having any more surgery and wanted to know what her options were. After extensive testing and baseline studies, we started her on a strong program of cancer prevention, consisting of anti-aging nutritional supplements together with other lifestyle adjustments. The program was designed to keep her cancer in remission as long as possible. Hormone replacement therapy was out of the question due to her cancer.

After two months on our anti-aging program, she felt better than she had felt in years. Her cancer markers started to come down and they stayed low. Her oncologist was pleasantly surprised when MJ told him what she was taking. Indeed, individuals with cancer in remission can be ideal candidates for embarking on an anti-aging program. The body has already been injured, and despite aggressive surgery, chemotherapy and radiotherapy, chances are that some pre-cancerous or cancer cells remain. MJ was smart enough to know that. She did not want to take any chances. Enrolling on our program was much cheaper and more comfortable than undergoing surgery, and she was aware of that. That case took place over a few years ago and she remains in remission. In fact, her blood work, for a woman who has had extensive medical problems, is better today than her husband, who is considered "healthy" by normal blood test exams.

FREQUENT ANTI-AGING QUESTION

Q: Can I increase my growth hormone level without taking shots or pills ?

There are two forms of exercise that stimulate growth hormone release. Intense aerobic exercises results in persistent long-term release of growth hormone in the blood for up to two hours after you stop exercising. Resistance exercises like weight training of layer muscle groups cause the spurts of growth hormone releases from the pituitary gland.

GASTRO-INTESTINAL AND
LIVER HEALTH RESTORED

MP is a successful lawyer in his mid-50s. A relaxed person by nature, he is in a highly-stressed profession, with many court appearances, social events and demanding clients. At the time of referral to us, his cholesterol was 280, with poorly balanced total cholesterol to HDL cholesterol ratio. His triglyceride was also high. His liver enzymes were elevated from years of alcohol consumption. He was also having problems sleeping, with frequent awakenings in the middle of the night and being unable to go back to sleep. His bowel movements were irregular. He was often constipated. There were also frequent flatulence, which was very embarrassing to him.

After evaluation and baseline testing, MP was started on our anti-aging program, with emphasis on detoxification, gastro-intestinal health, stress reduction and immune enhancement to his liver. After just two weeks, he started having more regular bowel movements. His digestive system balance was regained within four weeks with enzymatic therapy. He was able to sleep through the night. Needless to say, his productivity during the day increased and he was indeed a totally new person. Unfortunately, he still continues to smoke, a habit which he has yet to kick. He has, however, stopped the consumption of all alcohol. After being on our anti-aging program, he wanted to stop alcohol consumption automatically as he felt so much better without it. **MP is a typical patient who is smart enough to seek help and started the process of rejuvenation.**

TAKEN OFF DIABETIC MEDICATION

LP is a 69-year-old male. He had a number of medical problems including diabetes, low energy levels, irritable bowel syndrome, indigestion, hypertension and cardiomyopathy.

His fasting blood glucose was 223 mg/dl and he was taking an oral diabetic agent. His growth hormone level (as reflected by IGF-1 laboratory studies) was also quite low (78 mg/ml). This is indicative of adult growth hormone deficiency problems. LP was taking many other supplements (about 30 bottles per month) in the attempt to alleviate his problems naturally. However, his condition became worse as he was blindly mixing and matching formulas.

He started on our anti-aging detoxification program to cleanse his digestive system and to get his body ready for absorption of nutrients. After two months of the anti-aging supplementation program, his fasting blood glucose improved to 184 mg/dl. Three months later, his fasting glucose was down to 130 mg/dl. He stopped taking his medication for diabetes. After one month on the growth hormone rejuvenator, his hormone level improved to 85 mg/dl.

LP is still on the our anti-aging supplementation program. After just four weeks on the anti-aging program, he reported that his general health had improved by 60%. He felt more energetic and his stress tolerance level had also increased. He was able to stop taking medication for his diabetes. He was able to sleep better and had a better and more positive attitude towards life. **LP is very grateful for his renewed and rejuvenated self.**

CHEST PAIN DISAPPEARED AFTER ONE WEEK

ED is a 74-year-old female. She had suffered a stroke and a heart attack. She had a balloon angioplasty and had since suffered angina (pain in the chest). In addition, she had no energy and was diagnosed with diabetes and high cholesterol. She had difficulty sleeping at night and had shortness of breath during extended walks.

ED was taking Procadia, Lanoxin, Lasix and aspirin for her heart condition and high blood pressure. She was also taking insulin for diabetes and a lipid lowering statin drug for high cholesterol.

ED wanted to be on a "nutritionally dependent program rather than a drug dependent program". She started on our anti-aging supplementation and detoxification program. **After just one week, she was sleeping better, had no more angina, and her shortness of breath was reduced.** Our anti-aging program was able to wean her off some of the medication for her other conditions. Her medical condition is serious and although she cannot be totally off drugs, she is thankful that her condition has improved drastically.

OFF CHOLESTEROL MEDICATION AFTER 15 YEARS

HS is a 49-year-old male. He had a history of very high cholesterol (330 mg/dl) and triglyceride levels (800 mg/dl) since he was 25 years of age. He had been told that it may be hereditary as his father also had very high cholesterol. He was given prescription drugs (Mevacor and Lopid) to help lower his cholesterol and triglyceride. However, after years on the medication, he did not see any improvement. In fact, the cholesterol and triglyceride level actually increased! In addition, his liver enzyme showed abnormal elevation due to the side effects of the medications.

Once started on our anti-aging supplementation program, he saw immediate improvement in his cholesterol and triglyceride. After 30 days on our anti-aging supplementation program, his cholesterol went down went down by 30% to 220 mg/dl and his triglyceride level came down to 400 mg/dl! After 90 days, he saw further reduction as his cholesterol returned to a normal level and his triglyceride level continued to decline. After six months, his blood level stabilized at 156 mg/dl for cholesterol and 190 mg/dl for triglyceride. Two months after starting the anti-aging program, HS was able to stop taking his medication altogether. Without drugs, his liver function improved. He experienced no side effects from our natural anti-aging supplementation program.

He had definitely recognized a beneficial change in his eating habits as his appetite for sugary and salty foods have diminished. In addition, **he lost 16 pounds over the five months on our anti-aging program**. HS not only feels better, but more importantly, his risk for cardiovascular disease has been drastically reduced.

HORMONAL IMBALANCE

MN is a 44-year-old female. She experienced frequent headaches and pain in her left breast, which gradually became worse over four years. Her mammogram was normal. She also had high cholesterol 220 mg/dl (with 152 mg/dl LDL cholesterol and 55 mg/dl HDL cholesterol). Other symptoms included irregular periods, moderate to severe stress, short-term memory loss, insomnia, thinning hair, severe reduction in libido and vaginal dryness, and stiff joints (especially in the hands).

Since the age of 40, she had noticed a reduction in muscle strength and an increase in body fat (she gained 30 pounds over this four-year period) and wrinkles, and the onset of depression. She showed signs of multiple hormones related insufficiency syndrome (IGF-1 level was 72 ng/ml).

Within three days of starting our anti-aging supplementation program, her headache stopped completely and her breast pain disappeared. Within one month, all her other symptoms improved by 80%. Most importantly, her improvement came about without the potentially harmful side effects of prescription medication.

ABLE TO WALK PAIN-FREE AGAIN

TE is a 74-year-old male. He was diagnosed with severe degenerative joint disease on the left hip and was scheduled to have total hip replacement surgery. He had not been able to walk without pain. He even altered his gait in an attempt to avoid pain. He was taking anti-inflammatory drugs to control flammation of his joints and to reduce pain.

After one month on our anti-aging supplement program, **his pain reduced tremendously and he stopped taking medication. Needless to say, he cancelled his total hip replacement surgery.** He was very grateful for his renewed freedom from joint pain and was amazed at how quickly and effectively his joint was rejuvenated through natural methods.

HIGH BLOOD PRESSURE, CHOLESTEROL, HORMONAL IMBALANCE

MP is a 68-year-old female with a long history of high blood pressure at 160-170 mmHg systolic and 100-105 mmHg diastolic. She took Norvasc and Tenormin for many years, but her blood pressure had never really decreased or stabilized. She had hypercholesterolemia and was taking Mevacor just to maintain a blood cholesterol level of 270 mg/dl. She also showed subtle symptoms of hormonal imbalance, such as a bloated stomach, hyper-pigmentation, vision problems, and irritable bowel syndrome. She was given Depoprovera and Premarin for low estrogen level by other doctors prior to seeing us.

She gradually adopted our anti-aging program. In just two months, **her cholesterol was lowered to 160 mg/dl on the all-natural supplements.** She also stopped taking Mevacor. Her blood pressure was stabilized and came down to 140/90 mmHg after six months. After nine months, the medication for her high blood pressure was tapered off completely. With our anti-aging program, her symptoms of hormonal imbalance diminished.

CONCLUSION

These are just some of the many success stories of people who had real problems.

We do not have a magic wand and we do not promise a magical cure for all your diseases. Your individual response is determined by your genes, the degree of damage you had already suffered and how determined you are in following our anti-aging program.

The majority of who followed our program have improved. They are happier, stronger and feel younger. Many of them are able to get off medication and have a new lease of life free from pain and suffering.

FREQUENT ANTI-AGING QUESTION

Q: How is adult growth hormone deficiency determined ?

Determination takes the form of a complete history and physical examination, together with laboratory studies in the form of a spot or provocative blood and urine test. Laboratory studies measure the IGF-1 level as a surrogate for circulating growth hormone level. An IGF-1 level of under 350 ng/ml in an adult is considered evidence of deficiency, even though the level may be normal for the age group concerned. Between 20 to 40 years old, less than 5% of healthy men have less than 350 ng/ml of IGF-1. Starting at age 40 and especially by the age of 60, most of the adult population, including those seemingly healthy, have IGF-1 levels below 350 ng/ml.

CHAPTER **FOUR**

ANTI-AGING NUTRITIONAL SUPPLEMENTATION

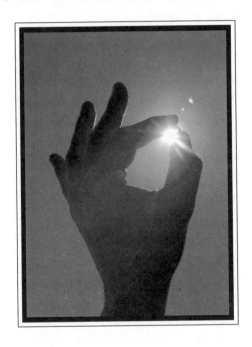

"I believe that you can, by taking some simple and inexpensive measures, extend your life and your years of well-being. My most important recommendation is that you take vitamins every day in optimum amounts, to supplement the vitamins you receive in your food."

Linus Pauling, PhD

INTRODUCTION

S upplementing your diet with optimum anti-aging levels of vitamins, minerals, enzymes and herbs **will significantly increase your life span**. These cannot replace proper nutrition but can aid in a healthy life extension. Not all nutrients are anti-aging supplements. Anti-aging supplements specifically address and prevent any possible deterioration in the cells that may accelerate the aging process.

The fact that supplements can aid in the prevention of certain diseases had not always been known. It was observed between 1500 BC and 1900 AD that certain foods prevented some diseases. For example, Egyptians used to take liver to ward off night blindness. From 1890 to 1900, the relationship between the lack of certain foods and diseases became established. The years 1900 to 1948 were known as the golden age of vitamin discovery. Many techniques for perfecting the production of vitamins, such as isolation and synthesis, were pioneered. In 1933, the first commercial synthesis of Vitamin C occurred.

Until recently, many fallacies existed about vitamins and minerals – do they really work? Do they not just go through the system and creates expensive urine? Are large doses dangerous? Should vitamins not be used only to prevent deficiency diseases, such as Vitamin C for scurvy and nicotinic acid for Pellagra?

Research has proven that optimum doses of vitamins are necessary for both the prevention of diseases and the promotion of optimum health. What constitutes "optimum doses" varies from very small to very large dosages, depending on the nutrients and the goal. Take Nicotinic Acid as an example: only

10 mg is needed to prevent Pellagra, but 1,000 mg is needed to prevent Chronic Pellagra. Another example is Vitamin C, where you only need 35 mg a day to prevent the onset of scurvy and 300 mg per day is needed for general well-being. For anti-aging purposes, 500 to 3,000 mg is recommended. For those stricken with cancer, as much as 50 gm is needed. The exact dosage depends on age, sex and the type of illness. Recent studies show that **vitamins also have important anti-aging effects that appear to be unrelated to their properties as vitamins.**

Recommended Daily Allowance (RDA)

Before advancing any further, a word on the Recommended Daily Allowance (RDA) is needed. The US Federal Government sets these levels. The RDA indicates the amount of vitamins and minerals needed to prevent common deficiency diseases (such as rickets or scurvy) for the "average person". The "average person" equates with that of an adult under 60 years of age, in good health, with normal digestion, with ideal body weight, leading a relatively stress-free life, with no medical problems, not in need of any medication and eating a balanced diet of 2,000 calories daily.

Needless to say, **most of us do not fit into this definition of the "average person". Even at the values set by RDA, most adult women do not meet the RDA for zinc, vitamin B, calcium, magnesium, or vitamin E. Likewise, most adult men do not meet the RDA for zinc and magnesium. Less than 29% of the US population consume five servings of fresh fruits and/or vegetables a day.** In fact, 20% of Americans do not eat **any** fruits or vegetables at all. Yes, they eat a lot of potatoes. While it is classified as a vegetable, potatoes behave like a sugar due to its high starch content. On top of this, older individuals generally consume less than 1,500 calories per day.

RDA of Vitamins and Minerals

RDA for Fat Soluble Vitamins:
- Vitamin A – 3,000 IU
- Vitamin D – 200 IU
- Vitamin E – 15 IU
- Vitamin C – 80 mg
- Vitamin K – 80 mg

RDA for Water Soluble Vitamins:
- Vitamin B1 Thiamine – 1.2 mg
- Vitamin B2 Riboflavin – 1.4 mg
- Niacin – 13 mg
- Vitamin B6 Pyridoxine – 2.0 mg
- Folic acid – 400 mcg
- Vitamin B12 Cobalamine – 3.0 mcg

RDA for Minerals:
- Calcium – 1,000 mg
- Magnesium – 350 mg
- Phosphorous – 800 mg

RDA or SAI (Safe and Adequate Intake) for Trace Minerals:
- SAI for Chromium – 50 to 200 mcg
- SAI for Copper – 1.5 to 3.0 mg
- RDA for Iron – 10 to 15 mg
- RDA for selenium – 75 to 250 mcg
- RDA for zinc – 12 to 15 mg

Is the RDA Sufficient for Anti-Aging?

In general, the RDA is inadequate if your goal is to retard or reverse heart diseases, cancers, cataracts, arthritis and other age-related diseases. For optimal anti-aging benefits, many health practitioners are recommending dosages many times higher than the RDA of certain nutrients. **Prevention of diseases requires that nutrients be on board at a minimum required level. Treating and reversing diseases require that these same nutrients in our cells be at a much higher level that can overcome free radical attacks and oxidative stress.** The cells must be well-nourished and armed with antioxidants well before the free radical attacks caused by poor dietary habits, pollution and stress set in.

Furthermore, ordinary serum blood tests are not adequate to reveal the true or functional level of each vitamin. **You can be "normal" based on blood levels, but actually lack the amount needed for optimum metabolic function, especially for anti-aging purposes.** To accurately measure the level of vitamins and minerals in the cells, ask your doctor to conduct a red pack cell study of these nutrients.

Some Alarming News

It is no secret that the diet for the majority of the US population is highly lacking in essential nutrients. You may feel full after a meal, but your organs are screaming for more nutrients. The longer you deprive your organs of the proper amounts of nutrients, the sooner you may see certain diseases and sicknesses set in. Nearly all **Americans are deficient in many nutrients, even according to the minimal RDA requirements. Half of all Americans over 60 years of age have Vitamins A, C, and E deficiency.** As we

---

FREQUENT ANTI-AGING QUESTION

Q: As we age, does our ability to absorb vitamins decrease?

Yes. As we age, our body's absorption of certain vitamins decreases. In particular, our body's ability to absorb Vitamin B6 decreases around the age of 40. In fact, many elderly people exhibit Vitamin B6 deficiency.

The body's ability to absorb Vitamin B12 also declines with age. Latest scientific studies recommend daily supplements of 500 to 1,000 mcg per day in order to counteract this impaired absorption in persons over the age of 60.

The brain's Vitamin B1 content also declines in tandem with the progression of aging and the body's requirement for Vitamin C increases. A daily intake of 1,000 mg of Vitamin C is recommended for anti-aging purposes.

---

age, our body runs out of steam. Our digestion and absorption of food is not as good, the production of hormones and enzymes slows down, and we have accumulated health problems. Much of this can be prevented with proper supplementation to the organs. Therefore, we need **more** nutrients. **Growing old itself can even be viewed as a vitamin deficiency disease of monumental proportion**. Worse, these deficiencies have been virtually ignored for the past century by traditional medicine. To add to this perplexity, we have learned that food cannot give us all the vitamins and minerals we need to slow down the aging process. Therefore, we are **all exposed to premature death**. The good news is vitamins and minerals for anti-aging are remarkably safe and free of side effects if taken as recommended. However, there is no one anti-aging miracle vitamin or mineral. They work together synergistically. In correct proportions and combinations, they support each other to counteract the aging process.

Optimum Daily Allowance (ODA)

The optimum daily allowance (ODA) represents a new reference level beyond the RDA which many researchers in anti-aging believe have cellular rejuvenation effects. These dosages are those frequently used in research studies and commonly practiced among those health professionals who believe that nutrition plays an important role in optimum health.

ODA is often many times higher than the RDA and for good reasons. To prevent diseases caused by deficiency of nutrients such as scurvy or rickets, RDA is prescribed. For optimum health and to prevent diseases such as aging or cancer, consider the ODA. It is that simple.

Here are just some examples of the differences:

Vitamin C: RDA is 85 mg, ODA is 250 to 3,000 mg
Vitamin E: RDA is 15 IU, ODA is 50 to 800 IU
Magnesium: RDA is 350 mg, ODA is 400 to 600 mg

The ODA is considered based on a completely healthy non-pregnant (also not trying to get pregnant), non-lactating adult who is not on prescription drugs and who intends to use nutritional supplementation to optimize heath and to prevent deficiency state diseases. Figures reflect a compilation of common intake levels among researchers and practitioners who focus on nutritional medicine as a way to promote better heath and longevity. These figures are not reflective of recommendations set by any governmental agency, as none exist. The exception is vitamin C and E, which the National Academy of Science has set as 2,000 mg and 1,500 IU, respectively, for the first time in the year 2000 as the recommended upper limit.

There is generally no benefit to consume amounts exceeding the ODA, except to treat specific disease conditions under expert medical guidance (eg. mega-dose Niacin for elevated serum cholesterol).

Safe Range

The Optimum Daily Allowance is well within the upper limit of many nutrients that can potentially cause side effects. While the ODA of vitamin A is 10,000 IU, safe range is up to 20,000 IU. Beta-carotene has been safely taken at dosage up to 100,000 IU a day, although the ODA is only 25,000 to 50,000 IU. Some may experience slight diarrhea or gastric discomfort after taking several grams of vitamin C, while others are not bothered by ten times that amount. While the ODA for vitamin E is up to 800 IU, one must be mindful that an intake of over 3,000 IU can cause headache, diarrhea, and increased blood pressure. Over consumption of magnesium in dosage of over 1,000 mg can lead to diarrhea that resolves when the intake is decreased. Rare liver problems have been reported in people taking Niacin of several thousand milligrams, while the ODA is only 25 to 100 mg. Calcium at up to 2,500 mg a day for long term use has minimal side effects, unless one has gastric ulcer. Excessive calcium unabsorbed can cause "milk alkali" syndrome.

Since each person is different, always consult a knowledgeable professional in nutritional medicine prior to embarking on any supplementation program designed for anti-aging and health optimization.

Precautions

While nutritional supplementation is generally very safe, those with specific health conditions should consult their nutritional medicine physician first to be safe. **If you are on a blood thinner, do not take excessive amounts of vitamin E, gingko or coenzyme COQ-10, all of which have blood-thinning properties. If you have kidney disease or heart failure, magnesium can exacerbate this problem. Zinc in high doses (over 300 mg a day) can inhibit copper, iron, calcium, and magnesium absorption. Those with Wilson's disease should not take copper supplements. Always discontinue all herbs and vitamins 1-2 weeks before surgery to avoid excessive bleeding from the blood thinning effects of many herbs and some vitamins.**

If you are of generally good health, taking nutritional supplements in optimum amounts should not pose significant health hazards.

Why Do You Need Supplements?

You simply cannot get enough of some of the vitamins and minerals in regular or anti-aging dosages even if you eat a healthy anti-aging diet (50% low glucose content fruits and vegetables, 20-30% protein, and 20-30% fat).

The following information on several important vitamins and minerals shows why food alone cannot provide you with sufficient vitamins and minerals to facilitate anti-aging.

1. Vitamin E – To get 400 IU of vitamin E, you need to take 28 cups of peanuts or consume 5,000 calories per day (and mostly in the form of fat).
2. Chromium – you have to consume 5,000 calories per day to get the minimum requirement of 50 mcg per day. **And to get the recommended 200 mcg of chromium for optimum health, you would need to consume more than 10,000 calories per day!**
3. Zinc – you have to eat 2,400 calories per day just to reach the minimum RDA requirement.
4. Magnesium – eating 2,000 calories per day is necessary to get enough magnesium in the modern day magnesium deficient diet.
5. Coenzyme Q-10 – you have to eat 1 pound of sardines to get 30 mg of CoQ-10 (healthy people need 30 mg a day for optimum heart function).

Aging is a disease accelerated by vitamin deficiency and malnutrition of monumental magnitude, which has been ignored for the past century. This silent epidemic affects 80% of all adults. Nutritional supplementation in optimum intake

levels is needed to ensure adequate levels for cells to carry out repair and rejuvenation processes.

The average American women lives to 79 years old, and men to 76 years old. The average person performs less than one hour of physical exercise a week and consumes an average of 2,000 calories a day. These calories are consistent with that found in fast-food restaurants – high in fat, refined sugar, low in fiber and low in dense carbohydrates. **If you want to live an average life, follow what the average person does. If you want to live longer and healthier, well into your 80s and 90s, the reality is that you have to do things that the "average" person does not do.** It is quite simple.

Study after study over the past 40 years confirm the fact that nutritional supplementation is a cheap insurance for longevity and cancer prevention if taken at the optimum dosage. **Nutritional supplementation is about food. It is not about giving your body something that your body does not have. It is to supplement your body's existing nutrient levels and to ensure that it is available for the body at all times.**

It is an accepted fact that people have different nutritional needs based on genetics, weight, gender, age, health status, the level of physical activity and the ability to absorb nutrients. **If you do not know what you need, the safest strategy is to err on the side of slight excess if you are in generally good heath. Having a little extra of any nutrient would not harm you, but a deficiency can lead to chronic diseases.**

Taking optimum amounts of nutritional supplements is a cornerstone and key component of any comprehensive

anti-aging program. You simply cannot get enough of these nutrients from your diet for optimum health. Having inadequate amounts over time can kill you. It is truly a "silent killer" over time.

CLASSES OF ANTI-AGING SUPPLEMENTS

Anti-aging supplements fall broadly into three major groups:

1. **Antioxidant Axis:**
   - Vitamin A
   - Vitamin C
   - Vitamin E
   - Selenium – a mineral
   - Magnesium – a mineral
   - Glutathione – an amino acid
   - Coenzyme Q-10 – a coenzyme
   - Chromium – a mineral that has hormonal enhancement properties

2. **Hormonal Axis:**
   - DHEA – a hormone
   - Estrogen – a hormone
   - Progesterone – a hormone
   - Testosterone – a hormone
   - Melatonin – a hormone
   - Glutamine – an amino acid with pro-hormone activity

3. **Specialized Function Axis:**
   - Bone Function – Calcium and Magnesium
   - Brain Function – Gingko biloba, a herb
   - Neurological Function – B Vitamins

- Brain Function – Phosphatidylserine, a fatty acid
- Prostate Health – Saw Palmetto, pygeum, stinging nettles
- Immunity Health – Zinc, a mineral
- Essential Oils

A note of precaution in relation to the consumption of some of these supplements:

- Magnesium – do not take excessive amount if you have kidney problems or severe heart failure.
- Gingko Biloba – do not take excessive amount if you have blood-clotting problems.
- Fish Oil – do not take excessive amount if you have blood-clotting problems.
- Niacin – liver toxicity in large doses have been reported.

If you decide to start on supplementation but have accompanying medical conditions, always consult a qualified health care practitioner before embarking on any nutritional supplementation program.

1. Antioxidant Axis

Just what are antioxidants? Specifically, they are chemicals that donate a sought-after electron to a free radical without themselves becoming dangerous. Excessive free radicals destroy our body and is one of the leading causes of aging. They are held in check by antioxidants. One trillion molecules of oxygen go through each cell every day, inflicting about 100,000 damaging free radical hits on our genes. Ninety-nine percent of these wounds are repaired by our body's endogenous antioxidants, but thousands of new wounds are left each day. By the age of 30, there are a few million oxygen lesions (wounds in every one of our body's cells). Scientists now postulate that it is this cumulative trauma that results in diseases such as cancer, stroke, and heart disease commonly found in the course of aging. **By the age of 50, about 30% of our cellular protein, especially in the arteries and heart, may be damaged by free radical attacks,** especially by molecules high in fat. Antioxidants prolong the integrity of our cells and, ultimately, our organs.

You may wonder where you can get proper antioxidants. They are available in healthy food and supplements. Fruits and vegetables contain antioxidants. **Astonishingly, eating five or more servings of fruits and vegetables daily will provide a large amount of antioxidants. However, most individuals do not eat the correct amount to slow down the production of free radicals. Supplementation is needed for most individuals, and certainly for combating anti-aging effects.**

Vitamin A (Beta-Carotene) — Fights Cancer and Heart Disease

Vitamin A is a fat-soluble vitamin that can be toxic in high doses. Beta-carotene is highly non-toxic and is converted into the productive form of vitamin A in our body. It is the smart way to take vitamin A.

Many studies have shown that people with high levels of beta-carotene in their diet not only have a less likely chance of developing cancer, especially of the lungs, but also of the rest of the gastrointestinal (GI) tract such as the throat, esophagus, and mouth. It takes at least 12 years of high doses of beta-carotene to thwart the onset of cancer of the lung. A large scale Harvard study of male physicians taking supplements of beta-carotene every other day for six years showed that the control group had only half the number of fatal heart attacks and strokes compared to

---

TOP 10 MARKERS OF HEALTH

1. **Body Weight** = ideal body weight less 5 to 10%.
2. **Systolic Blood Pressure under** 120 mmHg.
3. Percent **body fat** under 15% for men and under 22% for women.
4. **Bench Press** at least 50% of your weight.
5. Fast walk or jog at comfortable pace a **mile in under 15 minutes.**
6. **DHEA level** at upper limits for your age.
7. **Lipoprotein (a) level** under 14 mg/dl.
8. **Cholesterol level** at around 180 mg/dl, with HDL > 45 mg/dl and LDL < under 130 mg/dl.
9. **Serum ferritin level** at the low end of normal range.
10. **Serum homocysteine level** at the low end of normal range. (Target under 8 mg/dl)

---

the general population. **Another Harvard study of 90,000 female nurses showed that those taking the most beta-carotene (more that 11,000 IU per day) had a 22% lower risk of heart disease than those getting less than 3,800 IU per day.** In addition, the study showed that women who ate at least five carrots a week were 68% less likely to have strokes compared to the normal group. Eating a high volume of spinach also cuts the stroke risk by 40% (spinach has high content of beta-carotene).

The Alliance of Aging Research suggests that adults should take 10 mg (17,000 IU) to 30 mg (50,000 IU) per day of beta-carotene for life. One cup of carrot juice contain 24.2 mg of beta-carotene and one medium size sweet potato contain 10 mg. Incidentally, heavy cooking destroys beta-carotene.

If you want extra insurance against aging, many researchers favor a supplement of 15,000 to 25,000 IU of beta-carotene per day. Beta-carotene should be taken with meals because it dissolves in fat easily and increases absorption. Beta-carotene derived from a plant source is safe and non-toxic and a person can consume up to 100,000 IU per day.

Plain-type vitamin A, which can be found in most supplements, is derived from animal food such as liver and can build up the toxic level in your liver. Adults should take no more than 5,000 to 10,000 IU of this type of Vitamin A. High doses (more than 25,000 IU daily) of Vitamin A itself can cause hypervitaminosis, a condition characterized by yellowing of skin, blurred vision, loss of appetite, diarrhea and muscular weakness. These symptoms would disappear when the intake is decreased.

As far as antioxidants are concerned, both beta-carotene and Vitamin A are effective on their own. Together, their collective effect is greater. This synergistic phenomena is well-documented. In a Harvard study of female nurses, it was shown that there was a 34% drop in heart disease in those taking vitamin E alone; 22% drop in cardiovascular disease in those taking beta-carotene alone; and 20% drop in heart disease in those taking vitamin C alone. For those taking the highest amount of all three anti-oxidants, the rate of heart disease dropped by 50%.

Vitamin C — Good for Longevity

It has now been decades that the public knows the benefits of vitamin C. Dr Linus Pauling, a two-time Nobel Prize Winner, started taking high doses of Vitamin C in 1965. He died in 1994 at the age of 93. He believed that **his death was delayed by 20 years because of his Vitamin C intake. He took as much as 18,000**

mg per day in later years. In his work on vitamin C, Dr Pauling made it clear that he believed people could have an **extra 12 to 18 years of life** by taking 3,200 to 12,000 mg of vitamin C per day (equivalent to eating 45 to 75 oranges). Based on this hypothesis, he found in a study of 11,000 Americans that an intake of 300 mg of vitamin C per day (equivalent to five servings of fruits and vegetables per day) could increase an average of six years to a man's life and two years to a woman's life. Likewise, cardiovascular diseases in this group was reduced significantly.

It is interesting to note that animals (such as dogs and cats) that produced Vitamin C seldom get heart attack. Polar bears, for example, exhibit an average blood cholesterol level of over 400 mg/dl during hibernation and they seldom get heart attacks. Cardiovascular diseases on the other hand, affect over 50% of adults. Dr. Pauling postulates that this is due to chronic deficiency of vitamin C.

Vitamin C is a water-soluble antioxidant. Human beings is one of the few mammals that cannot produce Vitamin C and therefore must obtain it from external sources. Fortunately, Vitamin C is found abundantly in fruits and vegetables such as oranges, papayas, tomatoes and brussel sprouts. It's a supplement needed as an insurance against aging process.

Vitamin C also comes in a fat-soluble form called ascorbyl palmitate. Dr Pauling's studies had shown that when ascorbyl palmitate is absorbed, it fortify the micro-capillary wall of blood vessels that often deteriorate due to the aging process. His studies showed that when vitamin C is taken with the amino acids L-lysine and L-proline, there was a substantial reduction in atherosclerosis. A smaller dose of ascorbyl palmitate should be used because it cannot be flushed out of the system as quickly as the water-soluble form of Vitamin C. This allows more of the nutrient to get to and stay in the organs before leaving the body.

What Does Vitamin C Do?

Research on Vitamin C is so well-known that many people know at least two or three of its beneficial effects, which are wide ranging. It had been postulated to immunize against cancer, save arteries by driving up HDL and raise immunity by increasing production of lymphocytes. It reverses the biological clock by increasing the white blood cell level in the elderly, improve sperm and restore male fertility, combat gum disease, suppress high blood pressure and regenerate vitamin E and glutathione.

How Much Vitamin C Should You Take?

Normally, 300 to 1,000 mg is adequate for anti-aging purposes (note that one orange contains only 65 mg). If you take water-soluble vitamin C, you should take it 2 to 3 times per day for best results, as it is quickly flushed out of the body by our kidneys. If you are under severe stress, take up to 4 to 8 times more. The recommended dose for flu control is 1 gram per dose up to 10 grams a day. People with cancer may need to take 5 to 10 grams a day in addition to the intravenous vitamin C therapy of up to 50 grams each session in a course of treatment.

Side Effects of Vitamin C

In many studies, it was shown that there were no serious adverse effects from taking 10,000 mg of Vitamin C daily for several years. However, excessive amount may cause diarrhea, nausea and heartburn.

FREQUENT ANTI-AGING QUESTION

Q: How many vitamins and antioxidants should a person be taking for anti-aging purposes?

While the number of vitamins, minerals and antioxidants requirement for each person varies depending on the individual's needs, some generalizations can be made.

It is widely believed that "one-a-day" type of vitamins are insufficient for optimum health and anti-aging. A well-balanced, high-potency vitamin, mineral and antioxidant formula should be considered. Unfortunately, this requires many more pills (up to between 8 to 10). The key antioxidants should include vitamins A, C, E and Selenium. An intake of vitamin A in the form of Beta-Carotene (in the range of 25,000 IU), Vitamin C (1,000 mg), and Vitamin E (300 to 400 IU) is common for anti-aging purposes.

Certain minerals have also been found to have key, beneficial effects in anti-aging. This includes calcium (300 to 500 mg), magnesium (500 to 1,000 mg), and chromium (200 mcg). These minerals also have antioxidant effects.

To pack all the above nutrients into one single vitamin pill is impossible based on today's technology. Anywhere from 4 to 8 tablets is necessary to include all the above-mentioned key nutrients. Expect to take 30% more pills if the supplements come in capsule form versus a tablet form.

It has been reported to exacerbate iron toxicity in those with genetic disorders such as hemochromatosis. Those who have a sensitive stomach can take a chelated form of vitamin C, which causes less irritation.

Vitamin E — A Must-Take Vitamin

If there is a single most important vitamin to delay aging, many researchers and anti-aging physicians would agree that it is vitamin E. Vitamin E is a powerful anti-oxidant that fights atherosclerosis and cancer. You **cannot get enough of it from food,** unless you eat 5,000 calories per day (which would also have to be mostly fat). By the way, the RDA of Vitamin E is only 15 IU. **A suggested optimum dose would be about 400 IU** in order to prevent artery disease and oxidation of LDL cholesterol. The risk of not taking vitamin E may be equivalent to the risk posed by smoking, which we know can cause premature death. Vitamin E also prevents the clogging of arteries. Studies have shown that taking 800 IU per day for three months slashes LDL cholesterol oxidation by 40%. Likewise, in people over 60 years of age, taking 400 to 800 IU per day for 30 days result in improvement in immune function.

The recommended dose for vitamin E suggested by the Alliance for Aging Research is between 100 to 400 IU (the typical multivitamin carries about 15 to 30 IU). To get 400 IU per day from food alone, you would need to drink two quarts of corn oil, eat 5 pounds of wheat germ, eight cups of almonds or 28 cups of peanuts.

There are two types of vitamin E – natural and synthetic. The natural form is far superior in terms of absorption.

The most active biological form is alpha-tocopherol. Since vitamin E is a fat-soluble nutrient, there is a risk of toxicity to the system if taken in high doses. However, there is no significant toxicity up to 400 IU. 800 IU a day generally is a medically acceptable level. At this level, some blood thinning may occur. Therefore, higher dosages are not recommended for people on anti-coagulation therapy. At doses of over 3,000 IU per day, side effects such as headache, diarrhea, and increase blood pressure have been documented.

FREQUENT ANTI-AGING QUESTION

Q: How exactly can oxidative stress speed skin aging?

Wrinkles occur when the skin looses its elasticity. The loss of elasticity is caused by extensive formation and accumulation of collagen cross-links due to oxidative stress such as pollution or poor dietary habit. Another source of skin aging is sun exposure, which increases free-radical damage to the skin.

Selenium

This essential trace mineral has powerful anti-oxidant and anti-aging properties. It is an essential building block for the making of glutathione peroxidase. It is one of the most important enzymes to neutralize free radicals.

It is a fact that as we age, our level of selenium falls. Blood Selenium level drops by 7% after the age of 60 and by 24% after age 75. Worse of all, declining levels of selenium signify less antioxidant activity in our body. A decreased level of selenium is associated with higher incidences of heart diseases, cancer and arthritis. In addition, animal studies showed that selenium is able to block up to 100% of various types of tumors. A University of Arizona study of 1,700 elderly Americans showed that those with low levels of selenium were more apt to have polyps in the GI tract (33% compared to 9% in those with high levels of selenium). Another study (a Dutch study) of 3,000 older people showed that those on selenium supplementation had reduced risks of lung cancer by 50%. Likewise, higher selenium intake can lead to reduced risk of heart diseases. Selenium prevents platelet aggregation that normally leads to blood clots and block oxidation of bad cholesterol. A large-scale Finnish study showed that **those with very low level of selenium in their blood were three times more apt to die of heart diseases.**

Selenium can be found in grains, sunflower seeds, garlic, meat and seafood, especially tuna and swordfish. The Brazil nut contains about 100 mcg of selenium due to the soil in which it is grown. It is recommended that you take between 75 to 200 mcg of selenium per day for anti-aging purposes. Most common multivitamins do not contain that much selenium and, therefore, you would need to supplement with a separate selenium capsule.

Glutathione

Glutathione is a naturally occurring amino acid that is in food and manufactured by every cell in your body. It is a fact that glutathione blood level drops by 17% between the ages of 40 and 60. **Individuals with low glutathione levels are one-third more likely to have chronic diseases.** Many hospitalized patients with chronic diseases have a glutathione deficiency.

FREQUENT ANTI-AGING QUESTION

Q: Are there certain vitamins that should or should not be taken together?

The first that comes to mind is iron, unless in the ferrous state. It is an oxidant and, in general, should not be taken with other vitamins unless prescribed by a physician for medical problems such as anemia.

Vitamin C is best taken throughout the day in a divided dosage rather than a large dose all at once. Time-release vitamins may be an alternative.

Pregnant or lactating women should not take fish oil or Vitamin A, unless prescribed by a physician.

Vitamin D and magnesium should be taken with Calcium to maximize calcium absorption.

Where is glutathione found? It is found in vegetables such as brussel sprouts, cabbage, cauliflower, broccoli, and in fruits such as watermelon and grapefruit. Vitamin C and selenium boost glutathione levels.

Coenzyme Q-10

Coenzyme Q-10, also known as CoQ-10. It is an enzyme produced by the body. It is also found in seafood. Like many of the other nutrients we have discussed, it is an antioxidant. Starting around the age of 20, the production of CoQ-10 slows down. One startling investigation revealed that a diseased heart shows severe deficiencies of CoQ-10. Statin drugs commonly used to lower cholesterol also reduces the level of CoQ-10 in the body.

Nobody is yet sure exactly how CoQ-10 works. We do know that like vitamin E, it is a powerful antioxidant that stabilizes cell membranes. Research appears to suggest that it also energizes the mitochondria (the energy factory of the cell). It is highly concentrated in heart muscles, which require a lot of energy to maintain healthy pumping around the clock. It is not surprising to find that CoQ-10 fights cardiomyopathy and halts relentless oxidation of blood cholesterol LDL. In some countries, cardiologists prescribe high doses of CoQ-10 to patients with congestive heart failure. In Japan, more than 10 million Japanese take CoQ-10 as a prescription drug for cardiac problems.

Where to Find CoQ-10: Can you eat a pound of sardines every day?

CoQ-10 can be found in many different products such as fatty fish like sardines, organ meats such as heart, liver and kidney, beef, soy and peanuts. The recommended anti-aging dose for healthy people is 30 mg per day, especially if you are over 50 years old. You would have to eat 1 pound of sardines or 2.5 pounds of peanuts to get 30 mg of CoQ-10 naturally.

How much of this nutrient is needed for therapeutic purposes depends on whether you are healthy or not. For people with chronic disease, 50 to 150 mg is suggested. Those with severe cardiac conditions would need up to 400 mg a day. Take it with meals for better absorption. You can take the whole 150 mg at the same time. No divided doses is necessary. Vitamin E, selenium, and the B vitamins all enhance and boost the biosynthesis of CoQ-10.

Can you take too much of CoQ-10 so that it becomes harmful or toxic? Studies have shown that in normal subjects, no significant toxicity have been found in animals or human beings.

So far, it is currently considered one of the safest substances. There are reported cases of mild nausea. **Those who are taking blood thinning medicine should note that CoQ-10 have been found to have blood thinning properties as well and may potentiate other blood thinning drugs such as Warfarin or aspirin.**

Chromium

Chromium is a vital trace mineral that is found in low doses in certain foods. It comes in many forms, the most effective of which is Chromium Polynicotinate. **It enhances the action of insulin and reduces blood sugar levels.** Furthermore, it promotes a rise in DHEA, another anti-aging hormone. Chromium levels decline with each decade of life. At any age, one can take chromium to delay the onset of heart diseases and diabetes.

The overwhelming majority of Americans have a deficiency in chromium. To achieve the recommended anti-aging benefits of chromium, many researchers recommend taking 200 mcg a day. Insufficient chromium causes blood sugar levels to rise, affecting more than 16 million Americans who have glucose intolerance and or diabetes.

Chromium — How it works

When we eat food, the level of sugar goes up in our blood. Our body secretes insulin to help move the sugar into the cells for energy. As we age, our cells' ability to move the sugar decreases. In other words, the cells become insulin resistant. Our body reacts by producing more insulin. In the interim, our body is bombarded with sugar (found in almost every food source we eat), which is destructive and accelerates aging.

Chromium increases insulin efficiency so that less insulin is needed. The exact mechanism of this phenomenon is not fully known. If you eat sugary foods, you will need more chromium because molasses of sugar can destroy chromium. Getting 33% of your calories from sugar can cause three times the loss in chromium compared to eating 10% of your calories in sugar.

Unfortunately, food contains very little chromium. In the best anti-aging diets, there is only 24 mcg of chromium per 1,000 calories. Foods high in chromium include broccoli, barley, liver, lobster tail, and mushrooms.

Chromium Polynicotinate, the organic type of chromium developed by the US Department of Agriculture, is the best form as it is readily absorbed and used by the body. An adequate anti-aging dose is 200 mcg a day. For optimum anti-aging effect, some researchers are recommending 400 mcg a day. For diabetics or those trying to improve their blood sugar levels, more may be needed (results can usually be seen within a few weeks). In such cases, it is always advisable to consult your physician first. It is rare to find 200 mcg of chromium polynicotinate in a regular multi-vitamin, so it may be necessary to buy it separately.

HOW TO ADD **20** YEARS TO YOUR LIFE ...

Prevent Diabetes — Add 2.4 years

Adult onset diabetes (Type 2 diabetes) affects 16 million adult Americans. It is a prevalent medical condition among aging and overweight individuals. The diabetic patient is unable to effectively regulate his blood sugar level. **Adult onset diabetes can be reversed** by following these simple guidelines:

* Maintain an ideal body weight. (It is even better if you can maintain your target anti-aging body weight, which is 5 to 10% less than the ideal body weight).
* Avoid overly sugary, nutritionally empty foods (such as candy, soft drinks, etc) and grains.
* Take Chromium Polynicotinate to help balance your blood sugar level.

2. Hormonal Axis

Supplements within this category enhance our hormonal system and restore our hormonal balance.

DHEA (Dehydroepicaenoisic Acid)

DHEA can be considered the master steroid, as it is the most abundant of all steroids. It is involved in the manufacturing of testosterone, estrogen, progesterone and corticosteroids.

FREQUENT ANTI-AGING QUESTION

Q: I understand that the precursor of DHEA is pregnenolone. Do I need to take both?

It is often advisable to take both. While pregnenolone is the "mother" of DHEA, pregnenolone is also the mother of many other hormones as well. The amount of pregnenolone converted to DHEA is, therefore, small. If you are on a total hormonal replacement program, you should take both DHEA and pregnenolone, although the amount of DHEA can be lower.

In animal studies, it has been shown to prevent obesity, diabetes, cancer, autoimmune disease, stress, and infectious diseases. In other words, it is an all-round anti-aging supplement.

Optimum intake for anti-aging ranges from 25 to 50 mg per day.

Estrogen

Estrogen represents an entire family of female related hormones. Physicians commonly prescribe it to post menopausal women to combat symptoms of depression and osteoporosis. It has been used for many decades by millions of women around the world.

Estrogen reduces heart disease and controls LDL-cholesterol. It prevents the hot flashes and mood swings associated with menopause. Some studies have shown that it prevents heart disease and the rapid decline in bone density after menopause. It has a stimulatory effect on the human growth hormone (hGH).

The influx of environmental estrogen (also called Xenobiotics) have caused many women to exhibit an estrogen dominance syndrome. Symptoms include PMS, pre-menopausal symptoms such as bloating, hot flashes and depression.

Being a prescription drug, you would have to see a licensed physician before starting on estrogen. Estrogen replacement should be taken in conjunction with progesterone and only after a careful evaluation and scrutiny of the risks and benefits.

Progesterone

Progesterone is a precursor of most other adrenal hormones. It counters the effect of estrogen. Natural progesterone is often better than the synthetic kind, having fewer side effects.

Progesterone is a growth hormone stimulant. It promotes the breakdown of fat and has properties to protect against endometrial cancer when given with estrogen for ten or more days per cycle. Progesterone acts to built bones and protects against osteoporosis. It acts as a natural diuretic, restores and maintains sex drives, maintain thyroid hormone action for thermogenesis (fat burning) and helps to prevent breast and endometrial cancer. The standard physiological dose for women is 20 mg a day. In men, small doses of 10 mg per application help to increase libido, reduce hair loss and protect against prostate gland cancer.

Natural progesterone identical to that made by the body can be extracted from wild yam. This is very different from "wild yam extract" commonly sold in health food stores that cannot be converted into progesterone in the body. During the pre-menopausal period, natural progesterone cream should be used from day 12 to 26 of the month. During peri-menopausal period, apply the cream from day 7 to day 26. During post-menopausal period, apply the cream from day 1 to 25 of the month. Men can apply the cream everyday of the month to protect their prostate, increase testosterone level, and reduce estrogen in their body.

Testosterone

Testosterone is a male sex hormone. It decreases with age, starting in the mid-40s. By the age of 80, males have only 40% of the level that they had when they were 40 years old. The decline in testosterone level contributes to the "pot belly" and loss of muscle mass in middle-aged men. Testosterone replacement therapy (TRT) for men is as potent in its anti-aging effect as estrogen and progesterone are for women. TRT is given as intramuscular injections, suppositories or a patch to the scrotum. It is also available as micronized capsules or sublingual lozenges.

TRT is a potent stimulant of the human growth hormone. It saves bone for men affected with osteoporosis. Being a prescription drug, you must see a licensed physician before starting on it.

One of the side effects of TRT is a higher level of PSA (prostate specific antigen) and a rise in hematocrit. PSA is a marker of prostate health. Those on TRT should do a PSA test every six months and an ultrasound for prostate screening yearly.

Testosterone cream when applied in small doses by women has a stimulatory effect to enhance libido, memory and other anti-aging effects. A 1 to 2% testosterone cream is commonly used.

Melatonin

In addition to being a regulator of our sleep pattern, melatonin is a hormone with powerful antioxidant properties. It is secreted by the pineal gland (the timekeeper of the brain and controller of our circadian rhythms). Melatonin is an immune booster, cancer fighter, mood elevator, and a natural sleeping pill. **Dosage varies tremendously from person to person. While the "standard" dose commonly found over-the-counter is 3 mg, some people need only 0.3 mg while others may need much more to get a suitable effect. For many, a lower dose (0.5 mg) actually works better than the commonly seen over-the-counter 3 mg dose.**

Melatonin should not be taken by pregnant women or nursing mothers, women trying to conceive and people who are on prescription steroids. **To maximize the natural production and release of melatonin, sleep in a totally dark room. Even a small amount of light can reduce melatonin production by our body.**

L-Glutamine

Glutamine is a non-essential amino acid found in protein. It is considered to be the mother of all amino acids. It can be synthesized from a number of amino acids such as glutamic acid, valine and isoleucine. In times of stress and disease, the body cannot manufacture enough (such conditions include stress from exercise, such as weight training or severe burns). Under such situations, supplementation of glutamine can make a world of difference.

As an amino acid, it is a neurotransmitter in the brain and is essential for proper brain function. It is also an energy source for the brain. In higher quantities, it becomes a powerful antioxidant.

Due to its effect in promoting recovery and healing, it is commonly added to protein drinks used in muscle-building programs since it prevents muscle wasting by slowing protein breakdown. Those who are in weight training may need about 2 to 3 grams per day, or more right after an intense workout or before going to bed.

Anti-aging benefits of L-Glutamine includes:
1. Improvement of immune function, therefore preventing infection (infection can cause cellular damage and increased stress), thus slowing the aging process.
2. Helps overcome daily stress, therefore preventing oxidative damage that causes cellular destruction.
3. Prevents catabolic effect from cortisol, thereby preventing acceleration of the aging process.
4. Promotes extra release of growth hormone. Two grams of glutamine has been shown to cause a four-fold increase in growth hormone levels and therefore helps to slow the aging process.

3. Specialized Function Axis

1. Bone Enhancer – Calcium 300 to 500 mg and Magnesium 500 to 1000 mg.
2. Cerebral Function Enhancer – Gingko biloba, 30 to 60 mg.
3. Prevent Pseudo Alzheimer's Disease – Vitamin B-12, 500 to 1,000 mcg.
4. Fight Homocycsteine – Folic Acid 800 mcg, Vitamin B6 and Vitamin B12.
5. Cerebral Function Enhancer – Phosphatidylserine 100 to 200 mg.
6. Prevent Benign Prostatic Hyperplasia – Saw Palmetto 320 mg, stinging nettle, pygeum.
7. Immunity Enhancer — Zinc, 30 to 50 mg.

Calcium

Few people, especially women over 35, need to be told about the importance of calcium in their diet and that supplementation of this vital mineral is needed. Osteoporosis is one of the top killers for women and also, surprisingly, for men. A study by a French scientist of 3,270 women over the age of 80 taking daily doses of 1,200 mg of elemental calcium plus 800 IU of vitamin D, showed that they had 43% less fractures of the hip and 32% less fractures of the wrist, arm and pelvis, than those who did not. No matter how old you are, you need calcium.

Most Americans get only half the amount of calcium they need for anti-aging purposes. Unknown to many, calcium deficiency affects men as well as women. Less than 50% of children in the US get the recommended dietary allowance of calcium.

Fresh infusion of calcium in the diet or in supplements keeps bones young. Intake of calcium should start at an early age to maximize bone mass early in life and to minimize bone thinning later in life. Bone mass buildup occurs mostly up to the age of 25 and stabilized from the age of 25 to 30 before its gradual decline. It is especially important, therefore, to make sure that girls have sufficient calcium before puberty and throughout their young adulthood in order to build up their bone mass, which generally erodes later in life.

Calcium — How Much to Take?

From an anti-aging perspective, we do not recommend taking more than 500 mg a day in the form of a supplement (even though RDA recommends 1,000 mg per day). As you will see below, we strongly believe that magnesium is a much more potent nutrient against osteoporosis, compared to calcium.

Calcium is found in yogurt, milk, broccoli, tofu, canned sardines and canned salmon with bones. A glass of skimmed milk contains 300 mg, and a cup of yogurt up to 400 mg. The best choice of calcium is calcium carbonate or calcium citrate. Be sure to read the label – **calcium gluconate contains only 9% elemental calcium, whereas calcium carbonate has 40%.** Knowing this is important because you absorb 10 to 30% more from calcium supplements than from food, especially from calcium carbonate.

Please pay attention to the fact that calcium toxicity can occur. Too much calcium can cause constipation. To prevent this, drink lots of water and space the pills throughout the day. Do not take more than 500 to 600 mg at one time for the best absorption.

Magnesium

Magnesium (Mg) is a ubiquitous element in nature. Both plants and animals have an absolute requirement for magnesium. Magnesium plays a central role in photosynthesis in plants, and many of the metabolic reactions in animals.

Magnesium is a co-factor in over 300 enzymatic reactions in human beings. It is required for sodium, potassium, and calcium homeostasis as well as for the formation, transfer, storage and utilization of ATP (the energy currency in our body) at the cellular level. You cannot live without magnesium. The lower the cellular level of magnesium, the faster the disease states develop and the faster aging progresses.

The RDA for magnesium is 300 to 400 mg per day. Most American women get only 175 to 225 mg per day, and men 220 to 260 mg. To get enough magnesium from your diet, you would need to consume about 2,000 calories a day. Nuts, whole grains and legumes are high in magnesium.

Three Causes for Widespread Magnesium Deficiency

1. *Low Dietary Magnesium Level from the North American Diet.* In countries where a refined diet is the norm, such as North America, there is a universal deficiency in magnesium intake from the diet. Ninety-nine percent of the magnesium in sugar cane is lost when it is refined to white sugar. Eighty to ninety-six percent of magnesium content in wheat is removed when refined to white flour. Magnesium is not added back to the soil or to "enriched flour" after the germ and bran layer have been removed. Fifty percent of the magnesium may be lost during the cooking process into cooking water. The Asian diet, which is whole-food based, typically provides 500 to 700 mg of magnesium per day, while the Western diet provides one-third of that amount.

2. *Intestinal Absorption:* Consumption of soft drinks (pop or soda) decreases the body's absorption of magnesium. In the intestines, the phosphoric acid in soft drinks and the phosphates in baking powder combine with the magnesium to form magnesium phosphate, an insoluble precipitate that is excreted through the feces.

The typical high-dairy, high fat North American diet contains almost four times as much calcium as magnesium. This unbalanced ratio coupled with the high fat content tends to suppress magnesium absorption. **Excessive supplemental calcium taken to encourage bone growth in children and prevent osteoporosis in adults leads to a decrease in magnesium absorption.**

3. *Urinary and Fecal Magnesium Loss:* Magnesium can be recycled through the kidneys with a 95% recovery rate.

ACTION PRINCIPLE

The Right Thing

Success is about doing the right thing at the right time. Success is about doing what you know is correct even though the world may not have awakened to your wisdom.

When you restrict your calorie intake to enhance your longevity, this is the right thing to do.

When you do strength-training exercises to improve your muscle tone, that is the right thing to do.

When you take your supplements when others around you may differ, you know if they only knew, they would do it, too.

When you do the right thing, you feel good. When you feel good, you live longer.

However, alcohol promotes magnesium loss, as do diets high in animal protein, sugar, sodium and calcium. High blood levels of adrenaline and cortisol (hormones released during stress) cause serious urinary magnesium losses. Excessive noise and heat stress also promotes urinary magnesium losses.

Blood Test for Magnesium Level

Sixty percent of the magnesium in our bodies exist in our bones, 39% in our cells, and only 1% in the blood. **The correlation**

between blood serum magnesium and intracellular levels is poor. Total body magnesium levels may decrease 20% during a fast with no change in blood level. While a low blood magnesium level may correctly indicate serious disease, a "normal" magnesium blood level by a traditional laboratory test may exist concurrently with a deficit in intracellular magnesium. To accurately measure intracellular magnesium levels, one needs to do a red pack cell analysis. Unfortunately, this test is relatively expensive and not readily available. An inconvenient but accurate method to measure magnesium levels is by a 24-hour urine measurement for magnesium after intravenous magnesium loading. This is seldom done due to poor patient compliance.

How Much Magnesium Is Enough?

The National Research Council recommended minimum daily consumption for magnesium is 150 to 250 mg for children under 10 years of age, and 300 to 400 mg for adults. Current statistics show that **only 25% of the surveyed population has a magnesium intake at or greater than the RDA.** Almost 40% consume less than 70% of the RDA. It is fair to say that the majority of the North American population has a sub-optimum intake of magnesium.

The RDA for magnesium is about 2 mg per pound body weight. The American diet typically provides 1.2 to 1.5 mg per pound of body weight. **Many magnesium experts believed that an intake range of 2.7 to 4.5 mg per pound (about 400 to 700 mg a day) is optimum.** Some on the forefront of magnesium research are recommending up to 1,000 mg per day for healthy people using the clinical symptom of diarrhea as a target marker. Once the marker is achieved, magnesium intake can be reduced. Asians, for example, are already taking 3 to 4.5 mg of magnesium per pound of body weight in their vegetable-based diet.

Common Symptoms of Magnesium Deficiency

1. Musculo-Skeletal Symptoms: osteoporosis, chronic fatigue and weakness, muscle spasms, tremors and restlessness.
2. Cardiovascular Symptoms: atherosclerosis, cardiac arrhythmias, sudden death, and vasospasms.
3. Female Issues: PMS (Premenstrual Syndrome), eclampsia, fibrocystic diseases.
4. Psychiatric Symptoms: irritability, depression, and bipolar disorders.
5. Neurological Symptoms: migraine headaches, excessive noise, and pain sensitivity.
6. Endocrine Symptoms: insulin resistance.

Clinical Uses of Magnesium

Prevention and Management of Primary Post-menopausal Osteoporosis (PPMO)

The use of calcium supplementation for the management of Primary Postmenopausal Osteoporosis (PPMO) has increased significantly since 1987, the year when the National Institute of Health increased the recommended daily intake of calcium to 1,500 mg for prevention of PPMO. This recommendation was made in spite of the different conclusions made by some clinical studies presented in the same proceedings. Results of some of these controlled studies presented showed that there were no significant effect of calcium intake on mineral density on trabecular bone and only a slight effect on cortical bone. Since PPMO is predominately due to demineralization of trabecular bone, there is no justification for calcium mega-dosing in post-menopausal women. In fact, soft tissue calcification can be a serious risk factor during calcium mega-dosing under certain conditions.

Many in the forefront of anti-aging research believe that PPMO is predominately a skeletal manifestation of chronic magnesium deficiency, facilitated by estrogen withdrawal during the postmenopausal period. We believe it. **We suggested raising the RDA of magnesium to 1,000 mg/day and lowering the RDA for calcium to 500 mg/day. Our proposed daily intake for calcium would be more in line with the World Health Organization's "practical allowance" of 400 to 500 mg calcium daily for adults. Such a reversal of the magnesium/calcium ratio would most probably lower the incidence and prevalence of many other degenerative diseases as well.**

Gingko Biloba

Gingko or Gingko Biloba as it is commonly known, is a popular herb that comes from the Ginkgo Biloba tree, which is found growing throughout the world. It is an herb that has been used by humans for 5,000 years. It is the most popular prescription drug in Germany and France for symptoms of aging associated with deteriorating memory. In 1988, it was prescribed more than 5 million times in Germany alone. Not only is it used to improve memory functions, it also possesses properties which improve blood circulation.

Gingko Biloba — What it Does

Hundreds of scientific papers had been published on Ginkgo, confirming that **Ginkgo stimulates blood flow to the brain** by:

- Dilating blood vessels.
- Decreasing platelet aggregation.
- Being a powerful antioxidant blocking the oxidation of fatty cell membrane.

As a result, it improves cerebral vascular efficiency, memory and peripheral circulation in conditions such as intermittent claudication. In addition, Gingko has been shown to help slow Alzheimer's disease.

Gingko — How Much?

The usual dosage of Gingko is 30 mg one to two times a day for protective function and three times a day to improve symptoms. Be alert to the fact that it takes four to eight weeks to see any benefits, and those benefits revert back when intake is stopped.

Gingko is considered very safe among natural drugs. Some possible reactions include upset stomach, headache, and slight dizziness in elderly patients. Reactions can occur in dosages as little as 120 mg per day. Consult a physician before taking excessive Gingko, especially if you have blood-clotting or blood thinning disorders.

B Complex

The family of B vitamins consists of eight vitamins, all of which are needed by the human system to function properly. All B vitamins are needed to help cells grow and reproduce properly. This group of vitamins is commonly known as the B Complex. The following is a listing of these vitamins and the benefits they contribute to your health:

1. B1 (Thiamine) is critical for mental function and nerve growth.
2. B2 (Riboflavin) is required for cell growth and release of energy.
3. B3 (Niacin) is required for proper cellular functioning and reduces serum cholesterol levels.
4. B5 (Pantothenic Acid) breaks down fat so that it can be converted to energy and is needed for the synthesis of vitamin D, hormones, and red blood cells.
5. B6 (Pyridoxine) converts amino acid to protein and synthesizes enzymes and prevents heart disease.
6. Biotin breaks down fat, protein and carbohydrates into energy.
7. Folic Acid promotes cell growth and cell division. It also prevents birth defects and heart disease.
8. B12 (Cobalamine) converts carbohydrate, protein, and fat into energy. It also makes red blood cells and helps prevent heart disease. It is necessary of proper neurological function.

B Vitamins

From an anti-aging perspective, the most important B vitamins are vitamin B12 and folic acid.

Vitamin B12 — Facts

It should be known that most people get enough of B vitamins from their food with the exception of Vitamin B-12 and Folic Acid. **Over 24% of people between the ages of 60 to 69, and over 40% of people 80 years and older are deficient in vitamin B12.** This is due to a decrease in secretion of an intrinsic factor in our stomach necessary for vitamin B12 absorption. Another fact is that **lack of vitamin B12 causes pseudo-senility that produces Alzheimer-like symptoms. Many people probably do not realize that you can have a "normal" blood test and still have**

insufficient vitamin B12 to carry out metabolic functions. Vitamin B12 deficiency can also cause pernicious anemia.

Vitamin B12 can be found only in animal foods such as fish, chicken and dairy products. Vegetarians are also more susceptible to B12 deficiency.

B12 Supplementation

Supplementation of B12 is recommended as an anti-aging insurance, especially after the age of 50. A typical multiple vitamin pill with 6 mcg of B12 contains the minimum requirement to prevent B12 deficiency. However, in older persons, **up to 1,000 mcg can be considered for anti-aging purposes.** It is advisable to begin taking B12 supplementation when you enter the clinical phase of aging around the age of 45.

Folic Acid (Vitamin B9)

What does folic acid do? Well, for one thing, folic acid metabolizes homocysteine (high homocysteine levels triple your chances of heart disease) and keeps it in check. As a result, it protects you from heart disease.

If you get less than 350 mcg of folic acid, you are apt to have high homocycteine level.

A few facts about folic acid:

1. The average American over 50 years old takes in only 130 mcg of folic acid per day.
2. The less folic acid in the blood, the more your arteries are going to be narrowed and clogged.

3. Smokers need three times more folic acid to have the same benefits as non-smokers.

It has been discovered that folic acid preserves mental function as you age. People with low folic acid levels are more likely to have depression, dementia, memory loss and other psychiatric symptoms. Depression has also been relieved by as little as 400 mcg of folic acid in those with the deficiency.

Foods such as dried beans, spinach, citrus contain the most folic acid. It is interesting to note that your body absorbs and uses up to 50% of the folic acid in the food you eat. However, a supplement is recommended in order to afford added insurance and to make sure that homocysteine level is kept low. Generally, though, you can get enough folic acid from food. **A dosage of 300 to 400 mcg a day helps to depress homocysteine hazard, cancer threats, and reverse psychiatric disorders.**

PhospahtidylSerine (PS)

This fatty acid is a better version of Ginko Biloba and optimizes a variety of functions at the nerve membrane of each nerve cell. **PS provides metabolic support for memory, learning, and concentration and for the decline in cognitive functions that are well underway by the fifth decade of life.**

PS works by a totally different pathway compared to Gingko and N-Acetyl-L-Carnitine (NAC), which are also nutritional supplements with cognitive enhancing effects. Optimum intake of PS is 60 to 120 mg per day. Various clinical trials indicate that PS can help to improve.memory, learning, vocabulary skills concentration, mood, alertness and sociability.

FREQUENT ANTI-AGING QUESTION

Q: What supplements should vegetarians pay attention to?

A vegetarian diet is wonderful for anti-aging purposes, especially as one gets older. Nonetheless, a vitamin B12 supplement may be called for because only animal food such as fish, chicken, meat and dairy product contain this nutrient. At least 50 mcg of vitamin B12 per day is good for starters; 500 to 1,000 mcg per day in older people is more appropriate for anti-aging purposes.

Saw Palmetto

This herb has been shown by many studies to help relieve the common symptoms of benign prostatic hyperplasia (BPH), a common problem associated with most males over the age of 40 to 50, with symptoms such as frequency of urine, difficulty in passing urine and a decrease in the force of the urine stream. This is due to enlargement of the prostate gland pressing on the urethra.

Optimum intake of Saw Palmetto is 160 mg two times a day. Look for products that also include stinging nettles (a wonderful natural diuretic) and Pygeum. Pygeum is another herb that can relieve the symptoms of BPH. Studies have shown that these herbs work together synergistically and much better than any one on its own.

The active ingredient in Saw Palmetto is beta-sitosterol, which inhibits the conversion from testosterone to Dihydrotestosterone

(DHT), a much more powerful version of testosterone that may be responsible for benign prostatic hypertrophy and some form of prostate cancer. Evidence is indicating that estrogen dominance is also a strong causative factor in BPH.

Zinc

Zinc is a mineral produced by the thymus gland. This gland is the site for T-cell production and is large and robust during adolescence, but starts to shrink progressively after puberty. T-cell lymphocytes are responsible for fighting infections in our body. Without T-cells, our B-cells falter in their ability to make antibodies.

The following are a few facts about zinc. First, 33% of healthy Americans over the age of 50 have zinc deficiencies and do not know it. On top of this, over 90% of older healthy Americans have a zinc intake below that of the RDA. Furthermore, you need a daily caloric intake of 2,400 to get the RDA for zinc. Zinc can be found mostly in lean meat, seafood (especially oyster) and poultry. Cereals, nuts and seeds are also high in zinc, but they contain fiber that blocks zinc absorption. This is critical because absorption by our GI tract is drastically reduced by the age of 50.

What is enough? **A daily dose of 15 to 30 mg is enough to preserve the immune function that can become compromised due to aging.** For those over 75 years of age, up to 50 mg may be needed under the supervision of a physician. High doses can actually depress the immune system.

Where does this leave supplementation? Supplementation is recommended if you want to enhance your immune system. Zinc has also been known to increase testosterone level and have an anti-aging effect, especially on the male. **If you want to enhance the anti-aging effect, supplementation should be considered.**

Essential Oils

Essential oils (or fatty acids as they are commonly known) are indispensable for optimum function of the body. They provide the basic building blocks for the body's numerous enzymatic and hormonal function. They are also precursors to eicosanoids. Eicosanoids lower blood pressure, raise body temperature, modulate bronchial passages, and stimulate hormone production. Their production is highly dependent on dietary fat.

There are 3 essential oil families: omega-3s, omega-6s, and omega-9 fatty acids. Both omega-3 and omega-6 posses the strongest ability to generate eicosanoids. Omega-9s are weaker and not labeled as essential but are helpful. The common source of omega-9s is olive oil.

The secret to optimum health lies in maintaining the right balance between the omega-3s and the omega-6s.

Omega-3 Fatty Acid

Eating deep cold water fish like salmon and tuna, or taking quality fish oil supplements, provides a reliable source of omega 3 fatty acid. **There are 3 types of essential fatty acid found in omega-3 fats and oils. They are alpha-linolenic acid (ALA), eicosapentaenoic acid (EPA), and docosahexatenoic acid (DHA).**

When sugar is ingested, it is broken down into small molecules and is reassembled as fats called triglycerides. Too a triglyceride level is an independent risk factor for cardiovascular disease. Sugar also raises insulin. When too much insulin is circulating in the bloodstream, the triglyceride increase tremendously, with concurrent bad LDL cholesterol increases, and good HDL cholesterol decreases. EPA in particular has strong triglyceride lowering effect. Having an optimum amount of EPA (from fish oil) on board is clearly important for anyone with a high triglyceride level.

Unfortunately, **some people cannot take a large amount of fish oil (3-6 grams a day) supplement without a "fishy burp" and smell.** Fortunately, there is an alternative. Flaxseed oil is an excellent and important alternate source of ALA. In addition, the body will also convert flax oil's fatty acids into EPA and DHA, but the conversion ratio is low and takes weeks. While the flaxseed oil is remarkable in itself, the value of the entire flaxmeal must not be discounted. It is an excellent source of fiber and contains cancer-opposing compounds call lignans that deactivates the more cell-stimulating forms of estrogen and helps to modulate the undesirable side effects of menstrual cycle.

Omega-6 Fatty Acid

Now let us take a look at omega-6 fatty acid. Over consumption of omega-6 fatty acid is an important cause of premature aging, leading to a variety of chronic degenerative diseases. Not all omega-6 fatty acids are bad, however. Gamma Linolenic Acid (GLA) is an important good omega-6 fatty acid. Evening Primrose Oil (EPO) is a good source of linoleic acid. It also provides the important gamma-linolenic acid (GLA), the good omega-6 fat. The common notion that omega-3 is a good and omega-6 is a bad fatty acid must be dispelled. Omega-6, just like omega-3, is a much-needed fatty acid for optimum function of our body. **The problem of the modern day diet is that we simply take too much omega-6**

fatty acid (from sources like corn oil, sunflower, and safflower oil) in comparison to omega-3 fatty acid, causing an imbalance of massive proportion. While a good balance is 4 to 1 or thereabouts, most modern day diet has a ratio closer to 20 to 1 of omega-6 to omega-3 fatty acid or more.

GLA has a strong cholesterol lowering agent. Clearly it is important to have the proper amount of the good omega-6 fatty acid on board for its GLA content if your cholesterol level is too high. Good sources of omega-6 fatty acid includes evening primrose oil (EPO), borage oil and black currant seed. The later two provides 4 times more GLA than that supplied by EPO and therefore are more potent.

Our body needs a complete array of fatty acids in proper dosage and proper balance for optimum health. Those who are healthy should make sure there are enough omega-3 fatty acid on board to provide the important DHA and EPA that have triglyceride modulation properties, together with the right amount of omega-6 fatty acid to provide the important cholesterol modulating GLA on board. A series of properly formulated and balance essential oil supplementation capsule therefore forms the basic foundation of a comprehensive longevity program. Those with cholesterol challenges should add more GLA through Borage oil, and those with triglyceride challenge should add more fish oil. **Those who cannot tolerate fish oil should consider flaxseed oil instead either in capsule or in liquid form.** To get enough omega-9 fatty acid on board, consider using virgin olive oil in unheated form during the meal.

CHAPTER FIVE

NUTRITIONAL
SUPPLEMENT COCKTAIL

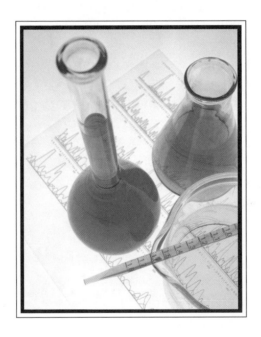

"Time waits for no one."

Anonymous

ANTI-AGING NUTRITIONAL COCKTAIL

The first and foremost step in an anti-aging supplement strategy is to choose a high quality, standard multivitamin/ mineral formula with optimum and safe levels of vitamins and minerals. While nutritional supplementation can be obtained "over-the-counter" and is considered a dietary supplement by the FDA, it is always prudent to consult your anti-aging physician for optimum dosage specific for your age, sex, and (especially) any associated medical conditions. Refer to the following quick reference guide for general **anti-aging optimum supplement strategy** recommendations for a healthy adult.

Antioxidant Axis:

1. **Beta-carotene (Vitamin A) – 10,000 to 25,000 IU**
2. **Vitamin C – 300 to 3,000 mg**
3. **Vitamin E – 100 to 400 IU**
4. **Selenium – 50 to 200 mcg**
5. **Magnesium – 300 to 1000 mg**
6. **CoQ-10 –15 to 60 mg**
7. **Glutathione – 50 to 100 mg**

Hormonal Axis:

1. **Chromium – 200 mcg**
2. **Estrogen – as needed**
3. **DHEA – as needed**
4. **Melatonin – as needed**
5. **Glutamine – 500 to 2000 mg**
6. **Progesterone – as needed**

Specialized Function Axis:

1. Zinc for immunity – 15 to 30 mg
2. Calcium/Magnesium for bone – 300 to 500 mg for Calcium and 500 to 1000 mg for Magnesium
3. Gingko for brain – 30 to 100 mg
4. Garlic for immunity – 3 to 6 capsules or eat lots of garlic
5. Vitamin B12 – 500 to 1000 mcg
6. Folic Acid – 300 to 400 mcg
7. Essential Oils – 1,200 to 3,600 mg

An individual who has serious illnesses (such as cancer) and wishes to pursue nutritional medicine as a way to overcome his/ her disease usually take a much higher dose as compared to the above. In cancer patients, for example, up to 50 grams (50,000 mg) of vitamin C is infused two to three times per week. The anti-aging doses mentioned above are far below the mega-doses some individuals are taking on an anti-cancer supplementation program.

A complete supplementation program requires the optimum dosage of almost 40 nutrients in a precise nutritional cocktail blend into 8 to 12 tablets/capsules. Is it really necessary to have a potent cocktail? The answer is "Yes" and there are reasons for it.

Why take a nutritional cocktail of over 40 nutrients? Because it works.

Here are the reasons:

First, different nutrients work on different parts of the cell. Vitamin C, for example, is water soluble and protects us from free radical attacks outside the cell. Vitamin E, on the other hand, is fat soluble. It is able to penetrate the cell wall easily and combat oxidative damage intracellularly.

Second, different nutrients complement each other in their duties. Numerous studies have shown that taking multiple nutrients in the optimum dosage is better than taking any single vitamin. There is no one single major bullet in nutritional supplement. It is wise to obtain as broad a coverage as possible.

Third, different nutrients have different target organs. Saw palmetto focuses on the prostate gland, while milk thistle focuses on the liver. Gingko has blood thinning properties and vitamin E improves circulation to the brain.

In addition to specific combinations and amounts of nutrients, a complete supplement strategy should take into consideration the age and sex of each person for maximum effect.

Age and Sex

There are inherent biological differences between men and women, which includes:
• Hormonal differences.
• Physical differences.
• Different external stressors.
• Different mental make-up.

For men, anti-aging supplementation should provide prostate support, increase immunity, preserve muscle mass and strength, and fight the cellular mutations that lead to cancer.

For women, anti-aging supplementation should support the hormonal system in pre, peri, and post-menopausal stages. Supplements for women over the age of 45 should be formulated with additional calcium, magnesium, folic acid and digestive enzymes (Amylase, Lipase, Lactase, Cellulase, Protease and Bromelain) to help enhance bone strength and promote healthy and strong skin, hair and nails. Herbs such as Valerian and Chamomile extract should be added to help the body cells handle stressful situations and produce a calming effect necessary for cell rest and restoration in the evening.

In other words, supplementation for women should be different from that of men.

Daily Body Rhythms

Your body goes through various phases during the day. To defend against daily stresses, you should take a nutritional cocktail that provides natural ingredients in the morning to energize your body and get you through the day. The evening intake should calm your body and prepare you for sleep and to rest and re-energize your cells.

FREQUENT ANTI-AGING QUESTION

Q: Is there any vitamin that people should take in addition to multi-vitamins with minerals if they like to eat desserts?

Chromium is one nutrient that dessert-lovers should take because sugar can destroy this trace mineral. Eating 33% of calories in sugar daily costs three times the loss in Chromium as compared to eating 10% of sugar in your diet. Surveys indicate that 75% of all Americans are deficient in the minimum recommended intake of Chromium (50 mcg a day). Many researchers are recommending 200 to 300 mcg per day. Those who do not get enough Chromium can have their insulin and blood sugar levels rise, causing diabetes and heart disease.

TOP 10 ANTI-AGING COCKTAIL INGREDIENTS

There are countless pills claiming they can help you to slow the aging process, but which ones really work? How do they work? Here are our top 10 favorites that you must have and should not go without.

1. Ascorbyl Palmitate/L-Lysine/L-Proline

- *Why*: This combination combats the number one killer of aging individuals – atherosclerosis, due to accumulation of lipoprotein (a).
- *How:* Based on research by Dr Linus Pauling, which conclusively links cardiovascular disease to the accumulation of plagues made of lipoprotein (a), and LDL, in the vascular wall. Human beings do not have the ability to make endogenous ascorbic acid (and therefore have a sub-clinical chronic ascorbic deficiency). This leads to the extra-cellular accumulation of LP (a) and fibrinogen/fibrin, the hallmarks of the soft atherosclerotic lesion that can result in vascular occlusion and heart attacks.
- *Dosage:* Ascobyl Palmitate 100 to 300 mg
  L-Lysine 150 to 300 mg
  L-Proline 100 to 200 mg

2. B Complex Vitamins

- *Why:* B Complex vitamins are one of the cheapest and most beneficial anti-aging nutrients. Many people will notice an improvement in mood, energy, alertness, concentration and memory when taking a good vitamin B Complex formula.

- **Diet:** Fast and refined foods decrease the amount of B vitamins in our food, particularly Folic Acid, B6 and B12, which are keys to lowering homocysteine, an amino-acid like substance known to accelerate hardening of the arteries.
- **Dosage:** Supplementation with 10 to 20 times the RDA of the B vitamins (which are water soluble and non-toxic) is recommended. Higher intake may be needed for those with medical, psychiatric or neurological disorders.

3. Garlic

- **Why:** Garlic has been used since ancient times and has been proven to have anti-bacterial, anti-viral and anti-fungal properties. Garlic also improves immune function, lowering of cholesterol, lowering of blood pressure, thus reducing chances of strokes and possesses anti-cancer properties. Garlic is an all-around herb for anti-aging purposes.
- **Dosage:** Take aged garlic of highest allicin yield (12,000 ppm) or one clove of aged garlic per day.

4. Coenzyme Q-10

- **Why:** CoQ-10 enhances energy production at the cellular level and is an excellent antioxidant. It is used clinically to treat congestive heart failure, coronary artery disease, high cholesterol level and high blood pressure (in high doses).
- **Maintenance Dose:** 30 mg per day.
- **Therapeutic Dose:** 350 mg per day.

5. Alpha Lipoic Acid

- *Why:* One of the most potent antioxidants that is both fat and water-soluble. It crosses the blood brain barrier to enhance brain function. It has been tested and shown to prevent a broad range of diseases, including diabetes and heart disease. There is not much in food and therefore supplementation is needed.
- *Maintenance Dose:* 50 mg per day.
- *Therapeutic Dose:* 300 to 500 mg per day.

6. Grape Seed Extract

- *Why:* Contains the bioflavonoid procyanidine (OPC) that is a strong antioxidant. It is responsible for the French Paradox where the French (who love to drink wine) have lower risk of atherosclerosis despite high intake of animal fat.
- *Maintenance Dose:* 30 mg per day.
- *Therapeutic Dose:* 100 to 300 mg per day.

7. PhosphatidylSerine

- *Why:* A phospholipid that is critical in maintaining the cell wall integrity of brain cells. Research has shown improvement in memory (far better than Gingko) after four to eight weeks of taking this. Also reduces blood pressure and cholesterol.
- *Dosage:* 100 to 200 mg per day.

8. Vitamin C

- *Why:* A potent antioxidant. It has well-proven clinical research as to its effectiveness. It helps lower blood pressure, possesses anti-cancer properties, reduces cholesterol and improves immune function.
- *Maintenance Dose:* 500 to 1,000 mg per day.
- *Therapeutic Dose:* 3 to 50 gm per day.

9. Vitamin E

- *Why:* A proven, strong antioxidant. It reduces heart disease, lowers cholesterol, alleviates menopausal symptoms, fights cancer, and prevents atherosclerosis.
- *Maintenance Dose:* 300 to 400 IU per day.
- *Therapeutic Dose:* 800 to 1,200 IU per day.

10. For Women – Magnesium
For Men – Saw Palmetto

Magnesium
- It is never too late to take Magnesium.
- Magnesium helps reduce cholesterol, lower blood pressure, improve brain function, and most importantly, helps prevent osteoporosis in post-menopausal women.
- *Dosage:* 500 to 1,000 mg per day.

Saw Palmetto
- Prevents Benign Prostate Hyperplasia. It is a must for any male aged 45 and above.
- **Dosage:** 160 mg standardized extract two times per day.

ANTI-AGING COCKTAIL –
THE DESIRED END RESULT

Eighty percent of us are going to die of cancer, stroke, or heart disease. Any effective anti-aging supplement program must address these three issues. In addition, the nutritional cocktail must fortify our immunity and modulate our hormones to deter the aging process. Initially, our patients are wary of taking supplements, especially when they are not used to it. The common program can range from 6 to 20 tablets, depending on the degree of anti-aging effect desired. In the end, the anti-aging nutrient cocktail works synergistically to achieve the following results.

Cardiovascular Protection – Our daily supplements must help to maintain the elasticity of the vascular system and help prevent cardiovascular complications. The following are key nutrients:

1. Ascorbyl Palmitate;
2. Vitamin C;
3. Vitamin E;
4. L-Proline; and
5. L-Lysine.

Cancer Prevention – Our daily supplements must contain antioxidants to help to prevent environmental free radicals to cause cancer. The following nutrients in optimum doses are required:

6. Vitamin A;
7. Vitamin E;
8. Vitamin C;
9. Selenium;

10. Grape seed Extract; and
11. Citrus Bioflavonoids.

Immunity Enhancers – Our daily supplement must help us to defend ourselves against germs, bacteria, environmental pollutants and external insults. Key nutrients in this area include:

12. Vitamin C;
13. L-Glutamine;
14. Garlic; and
15. Selenium.

Energy Boosters – Our daily supplements must provide natural sources of sustained energy throughout the day. The following are key ingredients:

16. Vitamin B12;
17. L-Glutamine;
18. Inositol;
19. Vitamin B6 (Pyridoxine); and
20. Vanadium.

Skin Rejuvenation – Our daily supplements must help to maintain the collagen of the skin and make the skin look and feel tighter and smoother. Important nutrients responsible for this include:

21. Ascorbyl Palmitate;
22. Vitamin C;
23. Calcium;
24. Magnesium;
25. Digestive Enzymes; and
26. L-Glutamine.

Hormonal Enhancers – Our daily supplements must help to maintain and balance the hormonal system. The following are key nutrients:

27. L-Glutamine;
28. L-Proline;
29. L-Lysine;
30. Evening Primrose Oil; and
31. Vitamin E.

Digestive Health – Our daily supplements must help to enhance the digestion and absorption of nutrients from food. The following are key nutrients:

32. Amylase;
33. Lipase;
34. Cellulase;
35. Bromelain;
36. Lactase; and
37. Protease.

Weight Management and Sugar Control – Our daily supplements must help balance our sugar level and prevent spikes that can lead to diabetes. The most important nutrient in this category are by far:

38. Chromium;
39. Vitamin C;
40. Vitamin E;
41. Digestive Enzymes; and
42. Vanadium.

How to add 20 years to your life ...

Prevent Cancer — Add 5 yrs

- Through early detection test.
- 90% of cancer is curable by catching it at an early stage.
- Supplement with a good antioxidant formula to help you protect your body from the free radical attacks that can lead to cancer.

NUTRITIONAL COCKTAILS FOR SPECIFIC FUNCTION

1. Improve Memory and Prevent Strokes

Helpful Nutrients
- **Vitamin B12** – to enhance neurotransmitter function.
- **Cats Claw** – to improve circulation.
- **Gingko Biloba** – to improve circulation.
- **L-Tyrosine** – to improve circulation.
- **Phosphatidylserine** – to enhance cell membrane stability.
- **Butcher's Broom** – to improve circulation.
- **Bilberry Extract** – to improve circulation.
- **EPA/DHA** – to lower blood viscosity.

What Do They Do?

- Help enhance short-term memory.
- Help improve thinking power.
- Improve the microcirculation in the neurological system.
- Protect against oxidation to cell by improving oxygenation.
- Aid people who have memory loss associated with Alzheimer's disease.
- Treat loss of concentration and emotional fatigue in adults and elderly individuals.
- Aid treatment of people who suffer from painful debilitating peripheral vascular disease, tinnitus and vertigo.

How Do They Work?

A lack of circulation or insufficient oxidation in our brain leads to early memory loss problems associated with Alzheimer's disease. The symptoms can be very disturbing and will cause changes in lifestyle or quality of life. The brain is the most important organ in our system – one out of four people die from stroke in the United States. This can also be categorized as the most debilitating disease once you experience it. The main side effect for stroke survivors is a lifetime of care. For those who have a history of strokes in their family or are trying to prevent it, taking the proper brain enhancing nutritional cocktail can help maintain proper blood microcirculation and help to prevent strokes.

The combination of Phosphatidylserine, L-Tyrosine and Gingko Biloba have been proven to help improve the blood circulation and the oxygenation in our brain vascular beds. These nutrients also help to increase circulation in the lower extremities as well.

The effects will actually generate healthier cells and possible rejuvenation of the already degenerated cells.

Many doctors and nutritionists also uses Omega-3 rich fish oil to help lower triglycerides and total cholesterol. Fish oil also increases HDL cholesterol which is known to help clear the plaques in the heart vessels. Fish oil, therefore, helps to mobilize atherosclerotic plaque from the brain's micro-circulation system, thus helping to prevent strokes.

Possible Interactions

There is no significant precaution needed, as these are food-based natural nutrients in a cocktail formulation.

Some of the ingredients have potential anti-inflammatory effects for arthritis and will improve the immune system as well.

Those who are already taking medication for stroke or other medical conditions such as Alzheimer's disease or memory loss syndrome, vertigo or dizziness need to continue taking their prescription drugs until the doctor advises otherwise. Do not assume that this is the immediate replacement of your medication.

Adjustment Period

No specific adjustment period is required.

Any allergic reaction to this combination of nutrients usually happens to people who have a history of allergies to a certain food.

Who Should Avoid This?

- Breast-feeding mothers.
- Infants and children.
- Individuals due for surgery (three to four weeks prior to the surgery, to avoid excessive thinning of the blood).
- Individuals with a bleeding condition.
- Pregnant women, unless approved by your health care practitioner.

2. Control Sugar Imbalance and Weight Control

Helpful Nutrients
- **Chromium Polynicotinate**
- **Vanadium**
- **Niacin**

What Do They Do?

- Promotes Glucose metabolism.
- Helps protein synthesis.
- Prolong the life of insulin, thus helping to regulate blood sugar.
- Helps to decrease insulin requirements.
- Improve the glucose tolerance in some people with adult onset diabetes.
- Helps to promote weight loss and increase muscle mass when used in conjunction with exercise.

How Do They Work?

Sugar is the first thing to avoid in preventing the acceleration of aging. Most Americans have a problem with "sugar craving".

Refined sugar appears in many of processed foods. This results not only in overweight people but also people who have the bad habit of adding refined sugar to their diet.

Most people do not have enough chromium in their system to facilitate sugar metabolism. When this happens, onset of adult diabetes (type 2) may occur. Even though poor sugar metabolism may not manifest itself in a form of a health condition, some people may suffer from swinging blood sugar levels throughout the day. This can cause personality or emotional disturbances.

Chromium Polynicotinate, a form of Chromium that is readily absorbed and utilized by the body, will help to regulate the body's sugar content. It helps to transport glucose into cells and enhances the effect of insulin in glucose storage and utilization.

Chromium also helps some people who are already taking hormones or drugs to maintain their blood sugar levels. When there is enough of this mineral in your system combined with other sugar metabolizing products, craving for sugar and sweets will actually stabilize. This will help the control of hunger pangs and eating habits. Further, controlling the craving for sugar will help tremendously in calorie restriction, which has been proven to prolong life expectancy.

How Much Do I Need?

The nicotinate form (Chromium Polynicotinate) has been found to be more effective than other forms. It is easily absorbed and utilized by the body.

For optimum anti-aging, the dose is 200 mcg a day. Those taking Chromium to balance blood sugar levels may need to take up to 1,200 mcg a day with other vitamins and minerals.

Those who abuse alcohol and drugs, have undergone surgery recently, are insulin dependent diabetics, have peripheral vascular syndrome and have numbness in the lower extremities due to problems with the vascular system may require a higher dose.

Possible Toxicity

Less than 1% of dietary Chromium is obtained from food. Therefore, it is very easy for someone to be deficient in this important mineral.

However, occupational hazards can occur to people whose jobs involve over exposure to tanning, electroplating, steel making, cement manufacturing, diesel locomotive repairs, furniture polishing, glass making, jewelry making, metal cleaning, oil drilling, photography, textile dyeing, and wood preservative manufacturing.

Possible Interactions

There is no significant precaution in this area, as it is a food-based natural nutrient.

Those who are taking prescription hormones (such as insulin) or medication for glucose problems need to continue with their medication. Always start slowly and on the approval of your private physician. Do not assume that this is the replacement of your medication. If you experience any improvement in your condition, your doctor may need to adjust your drug prescription.

Adjustment Period

There is no specific adjustment period required.

Any allergic reaction to this food-based nutrient usually happens to people who have a history of being allergic to Chromium.

Who Should Avoid This?

- Breast-feeding mothers.
- Pregnant women, unless approved by their doctors.
- Those who work in an environment with a high concentration of Chromium.

3. Boost the Immune System and Detoxify the Liver

Helpful Nutrients

- **Garlic** – possesses anti-viral, anti-fungal, and anti-bacterial properties.
- **Echinacea Extract** – enhances the immune system.
- **Milk Thistle Extract** – fortifies the liver.
- **Tumeric Extract**– possesses antioxidant and anti-cancer properties.

What Do They Do?

- Help to reduce the internal and external toxins in our body.
- Help to relieve cold and flu symptoms.
- Help with the wound healing process.
- Help to improve anti-tumor activities.
- Help to increase immunity.
- Help to improve recovery time after surgery or serious drug treatments such as cancer treatment.

- Help to protect the liver from chemical damage and help to treat chronic liver inflammatory disease (post hepatitis).
- Help to increase secretion and flow of bile.
- Possesses antioxidant effects.
- Help with indigestion.
- Help to improve urine production, thereby excreting excess fluids in the body.
- Act as anti-viral and anti-bacterial agents.

How Do They Work?

Echinacea (biological name *Echinacea angustifolia* and family name E Pallida) is a herb containing medicinal effect of the alkaloid, echinacoside, flavonoids, isobutyl amide, polkyacetylenes, polysaccharides and volatile oils. It is also called the natural antibiotic. It contains natural anti-toxins for internal and external infections. This herb improves the immune system and helps to fight the carcinogenic activities in our body as well.

Milk Thistle or *Silybum marianum*'s fruits, leaves and seeds are known for their medical uses as it contains the famous silymarin. Its chemical content is known to help reduce jaundice and inflammation caused by hepatitis, cirrhosis and gallbladder inflammation. Psoriasis patients report its benefits as well.

Garlic (*Allium sativum*) contains natural allicin, allyl disulfide, iron, magnesium, manganese, phytoncides, potassium, selenium, sulfur, unsaturated aldehydes, and vitamins A, B1 and C. All of these help lung circulation by decreasing lung mucous and improving the fluidity of the bronchial tubes in the pulmonary system. This promotes the control of blood pressure and can help to decrease cholesterol in males (reported in numerous literature).

Many people are using this compound to treat cramps, abdominal pain and even to inhibit certain forms of cancer. Some people may experience reddening of their skin due to improvement in blood circulation.

Possible Interactions

There is no significant precaution in this area, as this is a food-based natural compound. However, loose stool may develop during the first few days.

There are no significant adverse effects reported for pregnant or breast-feeding women. However, you may want to ask your health care practitioner if you are on special treatment or medication.

Adjustment Period

You need to consult your medical doctor after taking this for special conditions (such as the flu) or for other medical problems that do not improve within two weeks.

4. Protect Against Cancer and Oxidative Damage

Helpful Nutrients
- **Calcium D Gluconate**
- **Beta Carotene**
- **Vitamin E**
- **Vitamin C (Ascorbic Acid, Ascorbyl Palmitate)**
- **Quercetin**
- **Green Tea**
- **Grapeseed Extract**

What Do They Do?

- Act as powerful antioxidants.
- Help to prevent atherosclerosis.
- Prevent free-radical damage.
- Improve circulation.
- Possess anti-inflammatory properties.
- Help to protect against radiation.
- Help to prevent retinopathy.
- Reduce the risk of varicose veins.
- Help to heal wounds.

How Much Do I Need?

If you are in relatively good health, you need the following for general anti-aging health:

- Calcium D Glucarate – 50 to 100 mg
- Beta Carotene (Vitamin A) – 10,000 to 25,000 IU
- Vitamin E – 400 to 800 IU
- Vitamin C (Ascorbic Acid, Ascorbyl Palmitate) – 500 to 3,000 mg

If you know that you are more exposed to free radicals or other pollutants, you may wish to increase your intake. You should also review your intake with your healthcare professional if you had previously been diagnosed with severe aging conditions such as cancer or other malignancies.

Adjustment Period

No adjustment period required.

Allergic reactions to these food-based nutrients usually happen to people who have a history of allergies to certain foods.

Anyone who expects any change may feel minor symptoms such as dizziness or headaches (from possible increase in blood flow), occasional palpitation for those who have problems with conduction or even general restlessness. If these symptoms are from these nutrients, your body will generally adjust within one to two weeks, or three to four weeks at the most.

5. Reduce Joint Pain and Osteoarthritis

Helpful Nutrients
- **Glucosamine – rebuilds the proteogylcans, which form the cartilage structure.**
- **Chondroitin – helps to lubricate the cartilage matrix between joints.**
- **Bromelain – acts as an anti-inflammatory agent.**
- **Methyl Sulfonyl Methane (MSM) – a natural source of sulphur. It acts as an anti-inflammatory agent and provides pain relief.**
- **CMO**

What Do They Do?

1. Support healthy, mobile joint function.
2. Support connective tissues and bone.
3. Help to reduce the inflammatory effect and relieves pain from arthritis, over-exertion, and muscle fatigue.
4. Help to rebuild, lubricate and maintain the cartilage matrix between joints.

How Do They Work?

Pain is an "annoying" sensation that reduces one's quality of life. People will appreciate the effect when they are suffering from it. The combination of Glucosamine with Chondroitin promotes the manufacturing of GAGs (glycoaminoglycans) for optimum cartilage health and function. Bromelain is an effective proteolytic enzyme, which helps to reduce inflammation.

Glucosamine sulfate is a natural nutrient that has been the subject of more than 350 scientific investigations and more than 15 double blind studies.

The prestigious *Lancet* medical journal has published the most recent studies that created a new trend in treating orthopedic patients' pain with natural forms of medication, such as Glucosamine sulfate.

How Much Do I Need?

1,000 to 1,500 mg Glucosamine, 200 to 300 mg Chondroitin, 1000 to 3000 mg of MSM and 500 to 750 GDU Bromelain is good for optimum joint function and if you are in relatively good health. If you have severe joint damage, then you should increase your intake by two to three times. It may take 30 to 60 days before you expect to see any changes. If you do not experience any improvement within 90 days, the likelihood is that the nutrients are not going to help you.

Note: Smokers consume nicotine, thus decreasing the function of this combination of nutrients and its effectiveness.

Possible Interactions

There is no significant precaution in this area, as it is a food-based, natural compound.

Adjustment Period

No specific adjustment period required.

Allergic reactions to this food-based product usually happen to people who have a history of allergies to certain foods.

Who Should Avoid This?

* Breast-feeding mothers.
* Infants and children.
* Three to four weeks prior to undergoing surgery, to prevent impending clotting.
* Those with a bleeding condition.
* Pregnant women, unless approved by your health care practitioner.

6. See Better and Prevent Adult Macular Degeneration (AMD)

Helpful Nutrients
* **Lutein**
* **Vitamin A (Palmitate)**
* **Zeaxanthine**
* **Quercetin**
* **Bilberry Extract**
* **L-Glutathione**
* **EPA/DHA**

What Do They Do?

- Help to enhance eye health and visual acuity.
- Help to maintain the mucous membrane, thus preventing dry eyes.
- Help to improve the body's resistance, thus preventing infection and disease.
- Help to prevent cataracts.
- Act as strong antioxidants.

How Do They Work?

Vitamin A is essential for proper functioning of the retina. The red pigment of retina – opsin – forms the rhodopsin, which plays an important factor for sight in partial darkness. You have to be deficient in Vitamin A for many months before symptoms start to develop. Although the average person has approximately two years' supply of vitamin A in his or her liver, supplementation is necessary to achieve optimal anti-aging health, especially for antioxidant purposes.

If you have low calorie intake or your intake is low in nutrients, supplementation with vitamin A (in the form of Beta-Carotene or Vitamin A Palmitate) will balance the need for this ingredient to protect any irreversible damage to your eyes. Those who consume alcohol, drugs, have prolonged fever, are under excessive stress, undergoing surgery, have burns or injuries, or children with impaired immune system may require extra vitamin A for optimum eye health.

Lutein and zeaxanthine are two antioxidants specifically targeted for the eye and prevents oxidative damage.

Omega–3 Fatty Acids contain DHA (decosahexaenoic acid) and EPA (eicosapentaenoic acid). These are key ingredients that help to impede blood clotting and help the process of regeneration of damaged arteries.

Bilberry vaccinium myrtillus has been used and reported to help the treatment of diabetic retinopathy and cataracts. This plant contains chemicals such as anthoyayanins, flavonoids, hydroquinone, loeanolic acid and neomyrtillin.

How Much Do I Need?

5,000 to 10,000 IU of Vitamin A and 2.5 to 5 mg of Lutein is good to start with if you recognize the potential of having eye problems. You may increase your intake if your vision is sub-optimal.

Take it for at least 90 to 120 days before you review your test or expect any changes. Remember, these are natural nutrients. They will work, but not at the speed of synthetic drugs.

Safe Intake Range

Since vitamin A is fat-soluble, you should stop taking it if you develop any allergies. With natural based Beta-Carotene, there have been no reports of overdosage, except skin color change to a more yellow/orange color when the intake of Beta-Carotene is very high.

Possible Interactions

There is no significant precaution in this area, as these are natural, food-based nutrients. Those who are taking prescription medication for their eye problems should not assume that these nutrients are a replacement. This combination of nutrients may interact with antacids, neomycin, and mineral oil, which will decrease vitamin A absorption.

Adjustment Period

No specific adjustment period is required.

Any allergic reaction to this food-based product usually happens to people who have a history of allergies to certain foods.

7. Prevent Heart Disease and Maintain A Healthy Vascular System

Helpful Nutrients
- **Coenzyme Q-10**
- **Magnesium**
- **L-Carnitine**
- **Hawthorn Berry**
- **Lipoic Acid**
- **Ascorbyl Palmitate**
- **L-Lysine**
- **L- Proline**

What Do They Do?

- Help to oxygenate the heart cells.
- Help to reduce the soft and hard plaque build-up on vascular walls.
- Help to strengthen the collagen molecules of the vascular walls.

- Help to prevent heart attacks and ischemic attacks caused by microcapillary blockages and leakages formed daily in our vascular system.
- Help the mitochondria cells produce and preserve energy for the heart cells.

How Do They Work?

This combination of nutrients has been proven to help mobilize the "soft plaque" which contains the cholesterol deposit along the vascular wall, especially the coronary vascular system. This combination of nutrients acts like the HDL cholesterol to erode away the clog and leave the lumen clean and patent.

This combination of nutrients also helps to dissolve the hard plaque found in the vascular system. This plaque usually contains calcium deposits that can be visualized in ultra-fast computerized tomograms (CT scan) of the heart. The efficacy of this combination of nutrients has been proven by scientific research studies and has helped thousands of people to regain their healthy heart function.

This cocktail is good to add to any existing comprehensive anti-aging supplementation for people who have a strong history of or have already been diagnosed with cardiovascular disease.

How Much Do I Need?

30 to 120 mg of Coenzyme Q-10 per day, 500 to 1,000 mg of magnesium, 300 to 1,000 mg of L-Carnitine and Lipoic Acid is recommended for optimum heart health.

Take it for at least 90 to 120 days before you review your test or expect any changes. A much higher dosage is needed in a therapeutic setting.

Possible Interactions

There is no significant precaution in this area, as it is a natural, food-based compound. Those who are taking prescription medication for their heart problems should not assume that these nutrients are a replacement. Coenzyme Q-10 may have some blood thinning effect. Those who are blood thinners should consult your physician first.

Adjustment Period

No adjustment period is required.

Any allergic reaction to this food-based product usually happens to people who have a history of allergies to certain foods.

Naturally, you may expect a change in your already existing conditions when taking this combination. Anyone who expects any change may feel minor symptoms such as dizziness or headache (from possible increase in blood flow), occasional palpitation for those who have problems with conduction, or even general restlessness. If these symptoms are from any of these nutrients, your body will generally adjust within two to three weeks.

CHAPTER **SIX**

HEALING WITH DRUGS
OR NATURAL COMPOUNDS

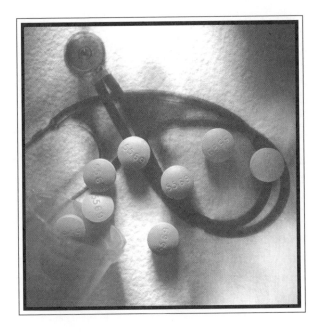

"Why kill a fly with a hammer?"

Anonymous

FREE RADICALS AND ANTIOXIDANTS

O ver the last 50 years, the concept of natural compounds such as antioxidants have arisen from hoax to science. It is now generally believed that **antioxidants have the ability to serve as a rust protector for the body,** putting a stop to a process called oxidation. Important molecules in the body, such as those that form the walls of arteries, become oxidized when they lose an electron. Once oxidized, they become unstable and break apart easily, leading to atherosclerosis.

The culprit is the free radical. Free radicals are highly reactive molecules or single atoms with unpaired electrons, looking for a mate to stabilize themselves. They steal an electron from the first molecule they encounter, perhaps a cell wall or a strand of DNA. Antioxidants are molecules that have extra electrons to donate to free radicals, thereby neutralizing them.

As free-radical damage mounts, cells can no longer perform at an optimum level. Tissues degradation begin and disease sets in gradually. An excess of free radicals is implicated the development of cardiovascular disease, Alzheimer's disease, Parkinson's disease and cancer among others. **Aging itself has been defined as a gradual accumulation of free radical damage.** By age 50, it is estimated that a large part of our cellular protein has oxidative damage.

Yet, not all free radicals are bad.

BENEFITS OF FREE RADICALS

Free radicals are necessary for life. The body cannot turn air and food into chemical energy without a chain reaction at the mitochondria involving energy production and free radicals as its by-product. Free radicals are also a crucial part of the immune system, attacking foreign invaders. They help fight against unwanted bacteria.

The production of free radicals and the destruction of free radicals in a non-harmful manner is also the result of normal metabolic processes in the body. Endogenous and exogenous antioxidants mop some of them up. **The body hopes to avoid excessive free-radical production, but a certain amount is absolutely necessary for life.**

POSITIVE STUDIES ON ANTIOXIDANTS

The job of antioxidants is to neutralize free radicals. **Studies have indicated fairly consistently that having too few antioxidants is bad for the body.** As early as 1983, a study published in the British medical journal, *The Lancet*, found that people with low blood levels of selenium were twice as likely to develop cancer compared with people with normal levels.

In the late 1980s, a landmark study, the Harvard-based Physicians Health Study – which had recorded the lifestyles of some 50,000 male health professionals for the past 15 years – found that men whose diet was rich in vitamins were half as likely to develop heart disease, compared to those with very low level of dietary vitamin E.

It is important to note that although these epidemiological studies suggest an association between antioxidants and good health, this does not mean that the antioxidants directly caused the improved health. Furthermore, it should not be concluded that taking antioxidants improve health without a concurrent healthy lifestyle.

Since the mid-1990s, numerous studies had suggested that nutritional supplementation commonly referred to as RDA (recommended daily allowance) should be increased. *The Journal of the American Medical Association* (JAMA) reported in 1996 that skin cancer patients given daily Selenium supplements were twice as likely to survive their cancer as those patients not given Selenium. This was a well designed, multi-center, double-blind, randomized, placebo-controlled study with more than 1,300 patients. The researchers were so impressed that the study was stopped after six years so that all patients could benefit with Selenium supplement.

Other studies showed similar positive results. Vitamin E has been shown to postpone the onset of Alzheimer's symptoms in a small study published in the *New England Journal of Medicine* (NEJM) in 1997. In 1995, *The Journal of the American Medical Association* (JAMA) published a report of a study conducted by the University of Southern California, School of Medicine. The study showed that vitamin E also slows down the onset of coronary artery disease. In 1998, a study published in the journal *Ophthalmology* reported that vitamin E also cut the risk of cataracts by 50%.

Vitamin C has its share of supporters as well. It has been shown to reduce oxidative stress in the retina and deter adult macular degeneration.

NEGATIVE STUDIES ON ANTIOXIDANTS

Over the years, various neutral and even negative reports about the benefits of antioxidant supplements have surfaced. One study found that Finnish male smokers were 18% more likely to develop lung cancer after taking a low dose Beta-Carotene supplement.

This was reported in *The New England Journal of Medicine* in 1994.

Three years later, *The Lancet* published a study of about 2,000 men receiving vitamin E alone, Beta-Carotene alone, both or a placebo after suffering their first heart attack. The group taking both vitamin E and Beta-Carotene was about twice as likely to die from a second heart attack or heart disease as the placebo group and the vitamin E group was about 1.5 times as likely to die.

Other studies showed similar negative results. A few reputable studies in the mid-1990s show no evidence that vitamins C and E or Beta-Carotene prevent the onset of colorectal cancer or atherosclerosis. There was also no evidence that Beta-Carotene alone prevented the onset of cancer or heart disease in more than 22,000 physicians over 12 years in one study.

Who is Right? They are All Right.

Criticisms naturally flowed back and forth, with the pro-supplement physicians finding methodological errors in the studies, while the anti-supplement wing found similar problems in the work that seemed to contradict their findings.

Most likely, all these studies may be absolutely right, pointing to the complexity of the matter – that we do not fully understand the intricate relationships between certain types of antioxidants and certain types of free radicals at different moments over the course of one's lifetime.

Each antioxidant is different. They work in different places, at different times and in different dosages. Blanket statements or broad conclusions drawn from studies from either camp will not stand up to scrutiny.

In the famous beta-carotene trial, where low dose beta-carotene is given to heavy smokers (whose body's cells are exposed from free radical damage and oxidative stress from the cigarette smoke and therefore cells are pre-cancerous), it is demonstrated that in fact, low dose beta-carotene increase the incidence of lung cancer. This is totally consistent with the fact that both cancer and normal cells strive in an environment of low dose antioxidant that is beneficial for all cell types.

Normal and cancer cell respond in the same way to low dose antioxidant therapy because both cell types require antioxidant in low doses for optimum function. In an environment of high dose antioxidant, however, the picture is quite different. Normal cells have mechanism to protect themselves when exposed to high doses of antioxidants while cancer cells do not. In other words, cancer cells have not yet adapted to the new insult and they suffer damage from the antioxidants. High dose antioxidants therefore selectively are toxic to cancer cells but not to normal cells.

It is important to take a step back and look at the whole process of oxidative stress in relation to the body as a whole for one to make sense of the conflicting reports that may surface from time to time.

The traditional cause-and-effect approach of medical and scientific studies work only marginally when baseline parameters of each antioxidant has yet to be formulated and verified.

Just as extra free radicals may be a detriment, extra amounts of antioxidants might be turning into pro-oxidants, fueling free radical production and its damage. In other words , too much of something may not be good. Animals, for example, produce vitamin C in an equivalent human dose of about 5 grams a day. This amount is increased by four times during stress. Humans do not make vitamin C. A reasonable dose of 1 gram to 3 grams a day is extremely safe and non-toxic. Most anti-aging researchers do not consider this amount excessive. Yet, in the lay community where the RDA is only 80 mg a day, the perception of taking even 1 gram of vitamin C per day may appear excessive.

Several studies have shown that people who did not get the RDA (80 mg) of vitamin C had an increase in free-radical damage to their DNA. Paradoxically, those who took mega doses (over 5 to 10 grams a day) of vitamin C also had an increase in DNA damage in laboratory experiments, although it is used as an anti-cancer therapeutic agent in selected cases. Compounding this is the fact that free radicals have been shown to kill certain cancer cells and can, thus, be good for the body.

Thirty years ago, our knowledge of cholesterol was quite limited. HDL cholesterol and LDL cholesterol had just been discovered. Their exact relationship is still unknown. Physicians were trained to lower the total cholesterol. Reduction of dietary cholesterol intake seems a logical and sensible approach. Today, we are aware of "good" HDL cholesterol and "bad" LDL cholesterol. More importantly, we know that it is the ratio of the good versus the bad cholesterol that is the key to optimum health and not the absolute total cholesterol level. We also know now that blood cholesterol level is more directly related to sugar intake than dietary cholesterol intake. Numerous studies have shown that the correlation between dietary and blood cholesterol level is only 15%. A similar story can be said about the good Omega-3 fatty acid versus the not so desirable Omega 6 fatty·acid balance which only 20 years ago was not known to the best nutritionist. The same can be said about the estrogen to progesterone balance rather than total estrogen alone as an indicator of hormonal health. The body is, indeed, the most miraculous machine on the planet.

Although the theory of free radical and oxidative stress was first advanced in 1956, we are still at the infancy stage in understanding it and the implications for anti-aging. Each study is trying to measure a specific parameter, but the very nature of the measurement is difficult to interpret due to our limited knowledge of how each vitamin works to begin with. **Researchers are often left with more empirical observations than logical conclusions.**

The danger lies in one trying to associate observations with conclusions. In the absence of better data, this is the best we can do, some researchers would argue. This is a normal process of any research, especially in a subject as complicated as this in its infancy stages. **The smart consumer and physician should take a global view of the entire body of research and its various observations and deduce an overall logical conclusion, rather than relying on any single research study to make any decision, as any such study at this stage of our limited knowledge is, by definition, imperfect.**

It should be clear that free radicals are as good as they are bad, and antioxidants in very high doses (higher than optimum doses) may do the body harm.

DRUG DEPENDENT OR NUTRITION DEPENDENT?

Which is the least riskiest way to the healing process and anti-aging? Is it safer to taking natural non-toxic compound such as antioxidants that is food based and that which has been clinically used and tested for centuries, or dependent on synthetic drugs that are recently developed in laboratory of giant drug companies?

Side-effect Statistics on Drugs

A recent study published by the Journal of the American Medical Association may shed some light on this. In this study, doctors are cautioned on starting their patients on newly approved drugs. **More than 10% of new drugs approved by the Food and Drug Administration (FDA) have serious side effects that are not discovered on initial testing and marketing,** according to researchers of the study, Dr Karen Lasser and Dr Paul Allen of the Department of Medicine at Cambridge Hospital in Cambridge, Massachusetts. In fact, researchers found that out of 548 drugs approved by the FDA from 1975 to 1999, 56 (10%) had to have a new "black box warning" indicating serious adverse reaction that may result in death or serious injury. Sixteen drugs (3%) were withdrawn, and 45 (8.2%) required one or more new black box warnings. Half of the withdrawals occurred during the first two years after the drug's introduction, and half of the new black box warnings occur during the first seven years. Therefore, **many drugs with adverse reaction went undetected until many years later.** One of the drugs, terfenadine (marketed in the U.S. as Seldane) was a popular non-sedating antihistamine. It was on the market for 13 years before being withdrawn because of arrhythmia. Another one called cisapride (marketing in the U.S.

as Propulsid) was available for 6 years before being withdrawn for similar reason. **The study found that the probability of a new drug acquiring a black box warning or being withdrawn from the market is a whooping 20% over a 25-year period.**

Drug Interaction and Overdose

Another example of a popular drug gone wary happened in August 2001, when the German Pharmaceutical giant Bayer AG withdraw the cholesterol-lowering statin drug Baycol from the market. This shocked the world. For years, the public is led to believe the wonders of statin drugs not only in lowering cholesterol but posses other health benefits as well. Millions of statin prescriptions are written yearly in the United States alone.

Unfortunately, Baycol usage was linked to 31 deaths. Moreover, deaths occurred at the manufacturer's recommended initial dose (0.4 mg/day) as well as at the highest dose (0.8 mg/day). The majority of deaths occurred in elderly patients and more often in women.

There are other statin drugs on the market, such as Lipitor (the best seller). Like Baycol, these drugs are linked to the same rare muscle weakness, known as myositis, which occurs in about 1 in 1,000 statin users. Myositis occasionally progresses to rhabdomyolysis – a complete breakdown of muscle cells that can lead to kidney failure and death. Some experts believe that pravastatin (Pravachol) and fluvastatin (Lescol) may have less potential for this deadly drug interactions. The data at this time are not sufficient to declare one statin drug safer or more dangerous than the others.

Drug interactions and side effects with statin drugs are not new. Numerous scientific literatures have reported adverse interaction including myositis when combinations of statins and other drugs, including warfarin (used to prevent blood clotting), clarithromycin (an antibiotic), and ketoconazole (an antifungal drug), are used. Laboratory test in animals have shown cancer development and liver damage when high dose statin drugs are administered.

The Baycol fiasco is just the tip of the iceberg, illustrating the growing potential for medical complications from drug interactions. Worldwide, doctors are increasingly relying on numerous pharmaceuticals to control chronic conditions, from elevated cholesterol to diabetes to high blood pressure and osteoarthritis. In about a third of the Baycol cases, deaths occurred among people who also took gemfibrozil (Lopid) – a drug used to lower triglyceride levels.

Most statin adverse effects, including the musculoskeletal (including rhabdomyolysis) and liver damage, are dose-related. That is, higher doses bring increased risks. Each doubling of the statin dosage also doubles the incidence of liver enzyme elevations that exceed three times the upper limit of normal. The Food and Drug Administration earlier reported 90 cases (63 confirmed) of liver failure and more than 30 deaths linked to statin drugs. For years, numerous researchers have been ringing the warning bell but were overruled. The public has been led to believe that side effects of statin drugs, if any, are minimal. Professionals are told that the benefits outweigh the risk.

What is the proper dose? Obviously, each person's dosage of any statin drug should be as low as possible to achieve the target LDL cholesterol. This is particular important for the elderly, women, and those of lighter weight. While seniors comprise only 17% of the U.S. population, they sustain 51% of the deaths from medication reactions. Studies have shown that up to 17% of all hospitalizations of the seniors are related to medication reactions. Often overlooked are women and certain minority groups such as Orientals who are smaller in size. Treating these with regular dosage could be a prescription for disaster.

According to the package insert of Baycol, the recommended initial dose is 0.4 mg/day. This dosage reduces LDL by 34% on average. But 0.3 mg – 25% less medication – reduces LDL by 31%. This target is sufficient for millions with elevated cholesterol to reach. No provision is made for those of different body weight, age, or gender.

Some doctors start patients at even higher doses than manufacturers recommend due to poor information. Product inserts of most statin drugs (including Baycol) do not include guidelines on how to titrate dosage based on the patient's weight and age. The lowest available dose of Lipitor, the best-selling statin in America, may be stronger than millions of patients require to achieve their target LDL cholesterol level.

Patients are treated like statistical averages, not like individuals – even when many individuals probably get better than average responses and therefore need only low doses.

The end result is over-treatment, which produces predictable and avoidable problems. Overuse of statin therapy was found among 69% of patients undergoing primary prevention and among 47% of patients undergoing secondary prevention in another recent article from *Journal of the American Medical Association*. Put it simply - over-treatment means increased, unnecessary risks for the patient. For some, especially those in compromised conditions, this may put them over the edge.

DRUGS VERSUS NATURAL SUPPLEMENT

Comparing the significant side effects of drugs to the almost **non-existence of side effect in natural food based compound with a negative risk of close to zero,** no wonder there is a worldwide trend in favor of using natural compound as the first line of defense against illness instead of drugs. The reason is simple – drugs are simply too toxic!

The rational physician should have a thorough knowledge of both drug based and non-drug based therapy, both for prevention of and treatment of diseases. Both options should be offered to the patient, together with the pros and cons of each. In both cases, the lowest rational dosing needed to accomplish the desired effect should be administered.

The question of whether to take supplements is an intellectual one. Doctors are divided on whether to recommend antioxidant supplements to their patients. The camp is divided into those who believe that there are not enough data to make blanket recommendations, and those who feel that most of us (particularly children) have such poor diets that they need a supplement to ensure an adequate amount for basic function, and those who say that anyone can benefit from more antioxidants regardless of how healthy the diet is. A smaller group sees the negative effects of antioxidants as reason enough not to recommend. **No amount of scientific data in the next few decades can convince the skeptical mind.** Our knowledge in nutritional medicine is growing exponentially. It is conceivable, though highly unlikely, that supplements might do nothing at all because they cannot get to where they are needed or because antioxidants might not be the magic chemical in the food we eat.

Whether to wait for more information, knowing that they will be conflicting from time to time, or to proceed with prudent and caution, depends on the amount of time left in one's lifespan.

Prevention of oxidative stress takes time, especially if one lives in a polluted environment. Aging is a process that starts around age 25. **When you are past the age of 35, you have entered the transition phase of aging and if you are past the age of 45, you have entered the clinical phase of aging. Taking optimum amounts (not mega dose amounts) of nutritional supplements should be considered seriously.**

The best anti-aging supplemental strategy focuses on the whole body. Fortify your body with the optimum amounts (not mega dose amounts) of antioxidants in accordance with the optimum daily allowance through a balanced nutritional cocktail as an insurance to maintain a proper balance with free radical productions if you are over age 25. As you get older, add nutritional supplements specific for your age, sex, and lifestyle. If you have specific medical challenges, consider nutritional supplementation as an alternative remedy if you are not keen on taking drugs.

CHAPTER SEVEN

HUMAN GROWTH
HORMONE (hGH)

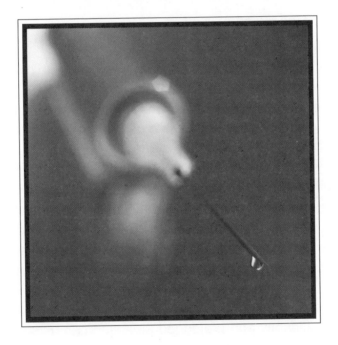

*"Old age must be resisted and
its deficiencies restored."*

Leroy "Stachel" Paige

Dr Ronald Klatz, world-renowned anti-aging expert, founder and president of the American Academy of Anti-Aging Medicine, states:

> By replenishing your supply of growth hormone, you can recover your vigor, health, looks and sexuality. For the ·first time in human history, we <u>can</u> intervene in the aging process, restore many aspects of youth, resist disease, substantially improve the quality of life, and perhaps extend the life span itself.

The American Academy of Anti-Aging Medicine, with over 10,000 health professional-members from more than 70 countries worldwide states that the **decreased production of human growth hormone in the body is a primary cause of aging.**

Work done in the area of growth hormone and the human genome is becoming well known and has been on the front page of virtually every major newspaper in the world. Can hormone replacement therapy extend the average life span? The answer is a decided **YES**. The reason we know this to be true is due to the successful experiments done by those involved with hormone replacement therapies. For instance, estrogen replacement therapy in post-menopausal women has reduced the rate of heart attack and stroke significantly and prolonged their life span. Research with human growth hormone (hGH) has been very encouraging because human growth hormone is pervasive in the body. Because of the exciting research and prospects relating to human growth hormone and aging, we are learning more about how this can help deter the aging process. Over a hundred articles published over the last 20 years and in the *New England Journal of Medicine* and other leading medical, scientific and research journals show that increasing human growth hormone may reverse human biological aging and make you look and feel younger.

HISTORY OF hGH

Human Growth Hormone was first discovered in 1912 by Dr Harvey Cushing. It was first isolated from human and monkey cadavers through glandular extraction in 1956. Two years later, it was being used to treat dwarfism in children by injection. In 1989, the landmark double blind study by Dr Daniel Rudman showed that with the use of hGH, **age reversal is possible.** This study included adult men who were tested for deficiency in growth hormone. These men were all between the ages of 61 and 73. They were injected with hGH made from recombinant DNA synthesis. In 1990, Dr Rudman's research results were reported in the prestigious *New England Journal of Medicine*.

Results of Dr Rudman's Landmark Double-Blind Study on hGH:

1. **Lean Body Mass**	**+ 8.8%**
2. **Bone Density**	**+ 1.6%**
3. **Adipose Tissue (Fat) Mass**	**-14.4%**
4. **Skin Thickness from 4 sites**	**+ 7.1%**

Summary: skin thicker, muscle mass increased, age-related stomach fat was disappearing, bone lost from the spine was restored.

FREQUENT ANTI-AGING QUESTION

Q: Is it true that you should not take hormone replacement on a regular and long term basis?

Our body has a built-in "negative-feedback" loop to signal the brain to turn off production of hormones when the amount circulating in the blood is too high. When you take external supplementation to boost your hormone level, the blood level rises and this feedback loop is activated. For this reason, most professionals recommend a resting period of a few weeks between cycles of hormonal replacement, including growth hormone and others. Interestingly enough, DHEA is not regulated by a negative feedback loop in the body. In other words, taking supplements of DHEA will not suppress your body's production of these hormones or cause the adrenal gland to rest, resulting in atrophy from the disuse. Theoretically, no "resting period" is required, although it may be a good practice to have a resting cycle of a few weeks for every few months of therapy, as with all hormone replacements.

The effects of just six months of human growth hormone therapy on lean body mass and adipose tissue mass were equivalent to **10 to 20 years of reversed aging**. Dr Robert Klatz's book *Stopping the Clock* says:

> ... it (human growth hormone) helps ... the way our muscle-fat ratio tends to change as we age. 80% of a young adult's body is lean body mass: muscles, organs and bones. Only 20% are fatty (adipose) tissue. For most people, after age 30, muscles atrophy, partly from genetic programming, partly from under use. Every decade thereafter an average of 5% of lean body mass is replaced by fatty tissue, so that by the time most of us reach age 70, we've gone from an 80-20 lean-fat ratio to a ratio that is closer to 50-50.

> The increase in fatty tissue is related to a variety of cardiovascular problems, whereas the loss of lean body mass is part of what causes the elderly to lose energy, strength, and mobility. Anything that can slow or reverse the trend towards more fatty tissue in effect slows or reverses the aging processes itself.

Although drugs and therapies that claimed to reverse aging are nothing new, only Dr Rudman's study passes the gold standard of drug testing: controlled, randomized, double-blind clinical study with reproducible results. **Dr Daniel Rudman's study in the *New England Journal of Medicine* at that time** represented the biggest breakthrough in anti-aging medicine and proved that certain parameters in aging could be reversed by 10 to 20 years!

Some of the most exciting and phenomenal studies in medicine today involve hormones and hormone replacement. For centuries, on all continents, humans have been practising medicine in a way which would prolong life. However, the scientific discoveries and development in hGH in this century has increased the possibilities of longevity to a qualitatively different level than ever before in human history. Clinical research in hGH expands with the passing of each year. Dr Rudman's studies in hGH defined a new era in anti-aging medicine. This is because **researchers can scientifically document that a substance can be administered to human beings that could produce age reversal.** Even before this study existed, the research into human hormones had been growing by leaps and bounds. Along with DNA research, hormone enhancement holds bright possibilities for extending life.

WHAT IS GROWTH HORMONE (hGH)?

Growth hormone is a small protein molecule containing 191 amino acids in a single polypeptide chain. It is the most abundant hormone secreted by the body in the pituitary gland. Its rate of production peaks during adolescence when rapid growth takes place. Release rate decreases 14% every decade. Generally, it remains in abundant supply in the pituitary gland waiting to be secreted into the body. For some cause yet to be identified, this all-important gland ceases to release the hormone into the body as we age and therefore fails to tell the body to repair the cells. By receiving decreased amounts of growth hormone over time, the body begins to age.

TOP 10 ANTI-AGING DO'S

1. Do **take your supplements** every day.
2. Do put yourself on a **good antioxidant program**.
3. Do consider **herbal therapies** to treat your ailments.
4. Do eat at least five servings of **fresh fruits and vegetables** a day.
5. Do incorporate **high fiber** into your diet.
6. Do eat lots of **fish**.
7. Do **exercise** regularly.
8. Do **relaxation** to reduce stress.
9. Do maintain a **positive attitude**.
10. Do visit your **doctor** for medical problems.

Daily secretion from the pituitary gland diminishes with age to the extent that from the age of 20 to 70, growth hormone level in your body falls by more than 75%. You look and feel older. Practically EVERYONE over the age of 40 has growth hormone deficiency.

Actually, secretion decreases due to lack of instructions from the hypothalamus to release growth hormones; receptor sites for hGH also become desensitized after a certain age. This causes less growth hormone to be released.

hGH is actually released in pulses that take place during the day, but are especially prominent during the beginning phases of sleep. The hGh is rapidly converted in the liver (within 20 minutes) to insulin-like Growth Factor Type I (IGF-1). More importantly, IGF-1 elicits most of the effects associated with growth hormone. It is measured in the blood and this is significant because it enables us to measure the amount of growth hormone being released. Many factors affect the body's ability to release hGH and form IGF-1. These factors include excessive physical and emotional stress, chronic liver dysfunction, poor diet, genetic predisposition and, of course, aging. Other factors leading to the decrease of hGH release include obesity, zinc and magnesium deficiency, an increase in blood sugar and/or insulin levels. On the other hand, factors leading to the increase release of hGH include calorie restriction, increased testosterone or estrogen levels, high doses of amino acids (L-Arginine, Glutamine, Lysine), increase in calcium and intense exercise.

SIGNS OF DECLINING HORMONAL HEALTH

The following are 15 common signs of declining hormonal health.

1. Do you go through mood swings easily?
2. Do you anger easily?
3. Do you have trouble falling or staying asleep?
4. Is your sex life declining?
5. Do you have problem concentrating?
6. Do you often get cold or feel sick?
7. Is your total blood cholesterol over 240?
8. Is your HDL cholesterol under 50?

9. Do you have high blood pressure?
10. Does the skin on your face and neck appear to hang?
11. Is it getting harder to exercise?
12. Is your grip strength weakening?
13. Is your endurance level less?
14. Is your breathing more labored when you exercise hard?
15. Are you age 45 and above?

If you answered "yes" to many of the questions, you should consider hGH enhancement.

EFFECTS OF hGH ENHANCEMENT

Reported effects with hGH enhancement are numerous. The loss of fat and reduction of wrinkles are reported as well as the growth of hair, better sleep, and increase in muscle. Improvement in sex drive, brain function, vision, immune function and cholesterol profile have been widely documented as well.

Three distinctive methods have emerged which either enable growth hormone to be replaced or stimulated.

The three methods are:

1.   direct human growth hormone injections;
2.   secretagogues; and
3.   hGH boosting hormone replacement.

The following is a brief summary on each of these categories:

Human Growth Hormone — Injections

For years after Dr Rudman's study, growth hormone was given by injection. Many inconveniences, however, sprung up as a result of using this method. Fortunately, these difficulties were not safety related but became, as we said, matters of inconvenience. For one, the injections were expensive and had to be supervised by a physician. Many people complained about having to poke themselves daily with needles. Besides the pain and inconvenience, people often had vascular problems associated with finding veins and new sites to inject. No major side effects were reported, with the exception of some minor joint aches and pains and fluid retention. This tends to disappear in the first or second month.

Although injections of human growth hormone may not be the program of choice for many people, statistics had shown the overwhelming impressive effectiveness.

A few years after Dr Rudman's death, a study was conducted at the same institution at which Dr Rudman had completed his original work. The following information was taken from this study at the Medical College of Wisconsin between 1994 to 1996.

Recipients of hGH were given low dose/high frequency dosages. The information was compiled from 308 randomly selected self-assessment questionnaires that were completed by 202 patients.

- **88% reported improvement in Muscle Strength**
- **81% reported improvement in Muscle Size**
- **71% reported improvement in Body Fat Loss**

- 81% reported improvement in Exercise Tolerance
- 83% reported improvement in Exercise Endurance
- 71% reported improvement in Skin Texture
- 68% reported improvement in Skin Thickness
- 71% reported improvement in Skin Elasticity
- 51% reported improvement in Wrinkle Disappearance
- 38% reported improvement in New Hair Growth
- 55% reported improvement in Healing of Old Injury
- 53% reported improvement in Back Flexibility
- 53% reported improvement in Sexual Potency/
  Frequency
- 73% reported improvement to Common Illness
- 62% reported improvement in Duration of Penile
  Erection
- 57% reported improvement in Frequency of Nighttime
  Urination
- 57% reported improvement in Hot Flashes
- 84% reported improvement in Energy Level
- 62% reported improvement in Memory

Findings such as these, which became nearly commonplace, began causing quite a stir in the medical communities, which resulted in a huge demand for human growth hormone for those who could afford and tolerate the daily injections. However, interest in being injected daily was not appealing to the mass public.

Most recently, researchers have therefore focused on methods that stimulate the pituitary to release the growth hormone, which is in storage but is not being released for some reason.

FREQUENT ANTI-AGING QUESTION

Q: What kind of diet is best for hormonal health?

A diet high in fruits and vegetables (complex carbohydrates) is best. Simple carbohydrates (such as cookies, rice, potatoes, and other sweets) increase blood sugar and insulin levels, which in turn decreases the formation of eicosanoids such as PGE1. PGE1 is a precursor to cyclic AMP, which is required for the production of melatonin, progesterone, testosterone, T4, and estrogen. Also required for the proper function of the growth hormone are ACTH, follicle stimulating hormone, luteinizing hormone, and TSH.

Nutrient supplements known to stimulate the production of hGH are called Secretagogues. In other words, these nutrients help the body to secrete existing hGH that are stored in the pituitary glands.

Secretagogues (hGH Releasers)

An unusual name: secretagogue (pronounced *se-cre'-ta-gog*). It is generally a natural peptide chain of amino acid that causes the pituitary gland to release the growth hormone, which has already been produced by the body and is stored in the pituitary gland. It is a food supplement and has no side effects. They are the precursor to hGH. While hGH injection cause the body to act as if the pituitary has released the growth hormone, a secretagogue actually causes the release of the body's human growth hormone. **Secretagogues do not act as growth hormones at all; rather, most of them stimulate the pituitary gland to secrete its own growth hormone.** Some advance secretagogue formulations stimulate the hypothalamus to release growth hormone releasing factor (GHRF) which in turn will stimulate the pituitary gland and release growth hormones.

Probably more than anything else, the inconvenience and unnaturalness of injecting hGH led to the discovery of secretagogues. For years, it was believed that the pituitary gland, where the growth hormone is produced, dries up as a natural effect of aging. Scientists had recently discovered that plenty of growth hormone resides in the pituitary, but that the pituitary merely stops secreting it as age progresses. The trick was to discover an agent, which could stimulate the pituitary to start secreting hGH again. Scientists discovered that certain combination of amino acids encouraged the pituitary gland to release the growth hormone. Experimentation had led to perfecting the right combinations.

How Does It Work?

A Growth Hormone Rejuvenator (secretagogue) will increase the growth hormone level. Research has proven that the human growth hormone declines with age. As it declines, we see the onset symptoms of aging. As the growth hormone level increases, many of these symptoms reverse and disappear. The growth hormone reaches far beyond the scope of many hormones to not only prevent biological aging, but to significantly reverse many signs and symptoms associated with aging. Reported effects of the increase in the growth hormone level are numerous. The overall feeling of vitality was reported along with a loss of fat and reduction of wrinkles with tighter and smoother skin, as well as the growth of hair, better sleep and reduced pain in joints. Improvement in sex drive, brain function, vision, immune function and cholesterol profile has been widely determined as well. There are a variety of secretagogues available. Unfortunately, many are not clinically tested. Our experience with selected oral effervescent and sublingual forms have been positive in increasing the IGF-1 level by up to 50 to 60%.

hGH Boosting Hormone Replacement

Certain hormones have a synergistic effect in boosting the body's secretion of hGH. Certain hormones, together with the growth hormone, decline with age as well. It is necessary to replace them to ensure your youth and health. Also, different hormones do different things in the body and raising the level of other hormones will decrease the amount of hGH needed. Some of these hormones are estrogen, progesterone, testosterone, DHEA and melatonin.

HOW NUTRITIONAL SUPPLEMENTATION AND hGH WORK TOGETHER

Following a good nutritional supplementation program, precision anti-aging exercise program, a healthy diet and the right mental health are vital because they work synergistically with hGH to promote hGH secretion.

FREQUENT ANTI-AGING QUESTION

Q: Other than getting injections, which is too expensive for me, are there any natural alternatives for me to increase my growth hormone level?

Many physicians practicing anti-aging medicine believe in using natural nutrients. It is done not by replacing the hormone, but by stimulating your very own pituitary gland to naturally increase the release of hGH. Substances, which stimulate the pituitary gland in this manner are called secretagogues. Secretagogues are all natural and side effects are rare. The results, while not as dramatic as injections, had been very encouraging.

In addition, **hGH can be enhanced with supplements such as Chromium Polynicotinate, which helps to lower circulating insulin and blood sugar. Finally, a natural hormonal enhancement program such as estrogen, progesterone, DHEA, testosterone, and melatonin can give an added boost to the secretion of hGH.**

Those over the age of 45 should consider hormone enhancement program. Secretagogues can increase your growth hormone level and the results could be dramatic, including loosing fat, smoothing wrinkles, increased energy, less pain and overall feeling and looking younger.

CHAPTER EIGHT

ANTI-AGING EXERCISE

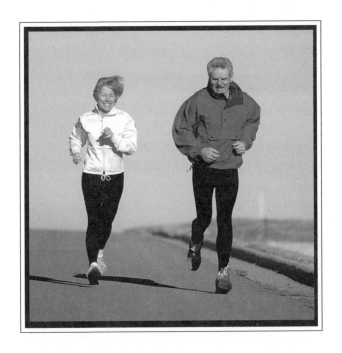

*"Life is 10% what you make it,
and 90% how you take it."*
Irving Berlin

INTRODUCTION

Y es, you have heard it before – exercise, exercise, and more exercise! Is it really that important? Why do you have to do it now? How much to do? What kind of exercise? What intensity?

If there is a magic pill for anti-aging, there is no doubt among leading researchers that exercise is it. Nothing comes closer to achieving anti-aging effects in our body than exercise. Research has repeatedly shown that those who exercise consistently live longer, happier and get sick less often. The bottom line is to do it or die!

From an anti-aging perspective, the real question is not whether to exercise but, more importantly, what kind of exercise, how much and how often. This is where the secret lies. To know the details is what separates the master from the amateur.

Anti-aging exercises consist of three separate components:

1. **Flexibility Training**
2. **Cardiovascular Training**
3. **Strength Training**

Make no mistake about it! Each of the components is equally important. It is well known that aerobics is good for the heart. What is less well known, but just as important, is that flexibility training and strength training contribute as much to longevity as aerobics. As you read further on, you will come to a better understanding of the reason. Suffice to say at this point that any anti-aging exercise program must be individually tailored to meet your personal needs, based on your current physical conditions. The program must also include, in a balanced fashion, all three components mentioned above.

Let us now look at each of the three components in detail.

FLEXIBILITY TRAINING

Flexibility training is the foundation of any exercise program because it increases blood flow to the muscles. It also warms up the key muscles of our body and allows your body to be more pliable and less prone to injury. Stretching only takes five to ten minutes a day. Think about it. The key to what you are trying to do is to have a healthy and active life. If you are injured, does that not defeat the purpose? **A simple stretching program before starting to exercise and during the cool-down period is, therefore, mandatory.** The lesson is simple: do not embark on any aerobic program or weight-training program without first doing stretching exercises for your key muscle groups.

CARDIOVASCULAR TRAINING

Cardiovascular (aerobic) exercise forms an important pillar within the entire anti-aging exercise program. It is one of the greatest anti-aging bullets available.

10 MYTHS ABOUT AEROBICS

1. **You have to work out at least 20 minutes to get cardiovascular benefit** — Long term follow up research has shown that life expectancy increases with consistent exercise, and that the difference between those who exercise ten minutes a day versus those exercising 20 minutes or more a day is the same. The key is to do it everyday.

2. **Low-intensity aerobics burns more fat** — Exercises at 60% of maximum heart rate causes the body to burn a greater percentage of fat as fuel rather than stored sugar (glycogen) or protein (muscle), but working more intensely at a higher heart rate (say 80%) causes more total calories to be burned, which is the bottom line in shedding body fat.

3. **Do aerobics first and follow it with weights to get lean** — Weight train first after a short warm up, then do cardiovascular exercise. This will conserve the energy you need to reach your target heart rate and will be closer to the fat burning mode desired in cardiac exercises.

4. **Aerobics is better than weight training for controlling body fat** — The best program utilizes both aerobics to burn fat (which is used for fuel) and weight training (powered by glycogen) to increase the basal metabolic rate by increasing lean body mass (for each pound of muscle mass, your body burns an extra 70 calories per day).

5. **Burn off extra desserts with another 20 minutes of aerobics** — A dangerous philosophy that sets yourself up for over training. If you must eat dessert, try to cut back on the amount and just work at a slightly higher intensity during the next few cardio sessions.

6. **Aerobics plus light weight lifting will lower total body fat without reducing muscle mass** — To alter the fat-to-muscle ratio in favor of muscle, you have to lift heavier weights to build up the muscle mass and, at the same time, do aerobics to reduce body fat.

7. **Eat a healthy meal to get the energy you need for aerobics** — For the first 20 minutes of aerobics, our body utilizes carbohydrates as fuel; thereafter, it uses fat as the fuel source. If burning fat is your goal, then loading up with carbohydrates is counterproductive. If you are running a marathon, then you need the extra carbohydrates to last as long as possible during the long run.

8. **Doing aerobics at lower intensity also builds heart health** — The heart is a muscle that needs to be stressed to be strong. The amount of stress depends on the physical condition of the person. Recent studies have shown that exercising 30 minutes a day, either in one continuous stretch or in blocks of 10 minutes each is equally beneficial. The key is to work your heart at 75 - 80% of your maximum heart rate.

9. **More aerobics is better** — Studies have shown that excessive aerobics (more than 3,500 kcal per week) flattens your longevity curve and leads to excessive oxidative stress. You should limit your aerobics workout to no more than one hour each session for optimum anti-aging purposes.

10. **Aerobics exercise benefits the heart only** — Research has shown that doing cardiovascular exercise at a heart rate of 80% of your maximum heart rate (calculated by 220-age) increases growth hormone release from the pituitary gland, which rejuvenates your body.

TOP 10 MOTIVATIONAL EXERCISING TIPS

1. **Understand** why you are doing it.
2. Set **realistic goals**. Anti-Aging is a marathon, not a sprint.
3. Find a **program that is right for you,** which you will follow and stay on.
4. Tell your friends and rely on them to **motivate** you.
5. **Visualize** what you can become.
6. Become a student. **Learn** as much as possible about your sport.
7. **Connect your mind and body**. Listen to your body.
8. **Reward** yourself, at least once a month.
9. **Define success** on your own terms – do not compare.
10. **Go slow, go steady – stay on course.**

The list of benefits from aerobic exercise resembles that obtained from growth hormone: gain of muscle mass and strength, loss of fat, increased energy, increased sense of well-being and a decrease in anxiety and depression. Moreover, aerobic exercise also increases the level of HDL-cholesterol, lowers blood pressure, improves the immune system and helps to protect the body against a host of chronic diseases, including cardiovascular diseases, stroke, hypertension, diabetes and osteoporosis. While research has shown that cardiovascular exercise increases longevity, the remaining questions still under research include: how much exercise is sufficient? How much is overdoing it? A famous study looked at 17,000 male alumni of Harvard University between the ages of 35 and 74. Results showed that as the physical activities of the men increased, the death rate decreased. **Men who spend at least 2,000 kilocalories per week doing moderate exercise such as tennis, swimming, jogging or brisk walking, lowered their overall death rate by 25 to 33 percent and decreased their risk of coronary artery disease by an astounding 41 percent when compared to their more inactive fellow alumni.**

The interesting new finding was that exceeding 3,500 kilocalories per week actually made things worse, giving a slightly increased death rate. The lesson to be learnt is that moderate exercise is the key to longevity, while extreme and over-exercise can lead to increased oxidation and tissue damage. Your heart may get a wonderful workout, but the rest of the body suffers tremendous damage from oxidative stress that occurs during extreme forms of exercises such as ultra-marathons (100 miles).

Those who do engage in such strenuous activities must take extra precautions to protect themselves from the excessive free radical damage that can occur from increased cellular respiration. Therefore, additional antioxidant supplementation is a wise choice for those who want to limit the amount of free radical damage in their bodies.

Cardiovascular exercise benefits any age group. However, it should be structured properly and should be scaled moderately to fit the particular needs of each person. You are advised to consult your physician to get medical clearance before, especially, if you are over 35 years of age.

How to add 20 years to your life...

Prevent Heart Disease — Add 9 years

Heart disease is the leading cause of death worldwide. Although there is a genetic component of cardiovascular disease, it is also a culmination of a lifetime of poor dietary and lifestyle habits. The following is a simple list of points to keep in mind to help prevent heart disease.

- Keep total cholesterol level between 100 - 200 mg/dl
- Keep LDL cholesterol under 150 mg/dl
- Keep HDL cholesterol above 50 mg/dl
- Three times a week of aerobic exercise, 30 to 45 minutes each time
- Strength training two to three times a week
- Yearly cardiovascular screening test after age 40

Maximum Heart Rate

From an anti-aging perspective, our goal with regards to cardiovascular exercise is to monitor the optimum point at which our heart is doing maximum work. **Because of age-related deterioration of the heart muscles, a young person's maximum heart rate is different from that of an older individual.** Fortunately, **the targeted heart rate is a relatively easy number to calculate based on the formula of 220 minus your age.** Therefore, if you are 50 years old, your maximum target heart rate should be 220-50=170. In other words, this is the maximum heart rate that you should generally not exceed, regardless of what form of exercise you take. If you happen to have a stress test by your cardiologist previously, you will realize and note that this is the similar number at which point your cardiologist will tell you to stop. **From an anti-aging perspective, we want the heart to be stressed but yet at the same time not over-stressed. Over-stressing the heart has certain advantages and disadvantages.** If you are young and training for competitive event, it is not unusual for the heart to be stressed to the maximum. During integral training, stressing the heart at maximum target heart rate would allow peak performance especially in sprint-type events where powerful burst of energy is required.

Intensity (Target Heart Rate)

The intensity of an activity can vary. Most anti-aging experts are in agreement that **between 60% and 80% of one's maximum heart rate is a good, reliable index of intensity.** If you are over 45 years old, over-stressing your heart can be detrimental to your heart. If you are 50 years old, your maximum heart rate is 220-50=170 beats per minute. If you take 70% of this then you arrive at 109, 80% of 170 equals 135. Therefore, if you exercise in an aerobic capacity which enhances your cardiovascular fitness, your exercise target heart rate should be between 109 and 135. This is, of course, a very general formula and does not apply to those who are training for competitive sports. As your cardio-fitness increases, your ability to train closer for maximum cardiac heart rate level will also improve automatically.

Duration and Frequency of Aerobics

Fifteen minutes of continuous or discontinuous aerobic activity on a daily basis is the minimum required for health and fitness. A better gauge is through measurement of calories expended, the ultimate standard in any aerobic exercise. Three to five times a week of aerobic activities is considered by most sport experts to be appropriate for the purpose of fitness. From an anti-aging perspective, your frequency is determined by the amount of kilocalories burnt over a one-week period. As we know today, **the optimum longevity burn rate is 2,000 to 3,000 kilocalories per week.** If you burn 1,000 kilocalories per exercise session, from an aerobic perspective, you need only two aerobic sessions per week to achieve this goal. The 2,000 kilocalories include calories burnt during strength training as well. So, weight training three times a week for 30 to 45 minutes a session accounts for 300 kilocalories per week.

This leaves you only 1,700 kilo calories to burn in aerobic exercise (three aerobic sessions of 500 to 550 kilo calories per session).

Aerobic Zone

For anti-aging purposes, the goal is to keep the heart in a healthy condition without over-stressing the cardiac muscles. For this reason, your exercise intensity should be adjusted so that your heart rate is no more than 60% to 80% of your maximum.

If you are training at 70% to 80% of your maximum heart rate, you are increasing your endurance capacity. In this zone, your functional capacity will greatly improve and you can expect to increase the number and size of the blood vessels to the heart, as well as increase your aerobic capacity and respiratory rate. At this level, 50% of your calories burnt are from carbohydrates and 50% are from fat and less than 1% is from protein.

If you are training at 80% to 90% of your maximum heart rate, you have entered another zone. In this zone, the exercise intensity is high and more calories are burnt per unit of time. Eighty-five percent of the calories burnt are from carbohydrates, 15% from fat and less than 1% from protein. For anti-aging purposes, it is not recommended that you remain in this zone for prolonged periods. A burst of exercise within this zone just to stimulate the heart and challenge it to meet adverse conditions on an intermittent basis (as in interval training) is acceptable.

Training at 90% to 100% of your maximum heart rate is not recommended for anti-aging purposes. In this zone, the highest number of calories per unit of time is burnt. Almost 90% of calories burnt at this intensity are carbohydrates. Only 10% are fat and less than 1% is protein. Very few people can last within this zone for more than a few minutes.

FREQUENT ANTI-AGING QUESTION

Q: Can over-exercise decrease longevity?

Over-exercising can have some negative effects on your longevity. A famous study of 17,000 Harvard alumni showed that those who exercised over 3,500 kilocalories a week had a slight increase in death rate as compared to the control group. Researchers postulated that over-exercise leads to an increase in cellular oxidation. This in turn leads to increased free radical formation, some of which can lead to cellular mutation and cancer.

FREQUENT ANTI-AGING QUESTION

Q: Why should you limit your cardiovascular training to 30 to 45 minutes per workout and not longer?

From an anti-aging perspective, the goal is to maintain our body at an optimum level of exercise as we age. It is not the design of an anti-aging program to prepare you for a marathon. Long training sessions, while good from time to time, can lead to excessive oxidation of muscle cells that in turn can lead to cellular mutation and cancer. Latest research has shown that cardiovascular benefit is evident after ten minutes of continuous aerobics exercise. In other words, you can break down your daily aerobic session into blocks of ten minutes each and still have cardio-vascular benefit.

STRENGTH TRAINING

There is no doubt among anti-aging experts that strength training should be an integral part of any anti-aging exercise program. The reason is simple: **your body mass decreases by 6% to 10% with each decade after age 30.** By age 70, you have only about 50% of our muscle strength left. Have you ever noticed how an elderly man shakes hands with you? The fact that the handshake is very weak is usually not because he does not want to shake firmly, but rather because the body's ability to affect a strong handshake is no longer there. Decrease in body strength leads to a decrease in body function, less energy, less balance and an increase in accident rate (the seventh leading cause of death among the elderly). Increasing strength, therefore, decreases the risk of accidents and increases longevity.

Exercise and Growth Hormone

Exercise, especially strength training exercise, sends a wake-up call to your pituitary gland to release growth hormone (growth hormone is a key anti-aging hormone). While the exact mechanism is not completely understood, properly performed anti-aging exercises stimulates growth hormone release, which has major significant benefits in increasing longevity. **If the large muscles group such as chest and back are involved, aerobic exercise have been shown to result in persistent, long-term release of growth hormone in spurts in the blood for two hours or even longer after you stop exercising.** Strength training also stimulates spurts of growth hormone to be released into the body as well. It is particularly interesting to note that while moderate intensity aerobic type exercise (60% to 70% target heart rate) is sufficient to cause maximum stimulation of growth hormone release. Weight training at 70% of maximum lift strength also causes a free-flow increase in growth hormone release. **At 85% of maximum lift capacity, growth hormone release into our body increases four-fold.**

FREQUENT ANTI-AGING QUESTION

Q: What is the single most important factor in an anti-aging exercise program?

The most important factor is consistency. If you cannot be regular with the program, it does not matter how great your exercise regimen is – you will fail. When you are busy, do less. When you have time, do more. Always do something to keep yourself in the program.

The Difference Between Anti-Aging Strength Training and Body Building

From an anti-aging perspective, the primary goal is to maintain muscle tone and muscle strength. You have the option of building muscle size for the purpose of entering a body building competition, if you so wish. Since the goals for anti-aging and body-building are different, the techniques and methodology are also different. From an anti-aging perspective, we want to achieve the following major benefits:

1. Increase in strength, decrease in accidents and increase longevity.
2. Increase lean muscle mass by replacing body fat to increase number of calories burnt even at rest.
3. Reduce depression and relieve stress.

Benefits of Strength Training

One important result of strength training is the increase in physical performance as measured by your strength. Stronger muscles enable you to lift and move things that are heavy. Stronger muscles also provide endurance regardless of what hobby, sports or day-to-day activities you engage in. From an anti-aging perspective, the primary goal is not really to increase the size of the muscle but, rather, to tone the muscle in such a way that the fat is replaced by the lean muscle mass. It is not unusual for those who are in a strength-training program to gain a few pounds of muscle as well as increase their strength and endurance by 30% to 40% after 10 to 12 weeks of consistent weight-strength training. This is achievable. A strength-training program changes body composition. An average 170 pound man with 20% body fat is carrying 34 pounds of fat and 136 pounds of lean body mass. After strength training, provided his weight remains unchanged, only 17% of his body weight is fat, which means he is now carrying only 29 pounds of fat, but 141 pounds of lean body weight. This change in body composition has a direct effect on the appearance resulting in a firmer look.

Strength Training and Metabolic Improvement

As we grow older, we generally lose about half a pound of muscle every year, which lowers our basal metabolic rate by about half a percent. A reduction in the basal metabolic rate means you need fewer calories to maintain your body functions so that your body converts less of the food you eat into energy. Instead, the surplus calories are turned into fat. This is the reason your body composition changes automatically as you grow older, even if you do not eat any differently. You notice that you are getting fatter and less muscular. This is the natural course of events if you do not do anything to counteract it. **If you are interested in maintaining the body composition you had when you were young, you have to be on a strength-training program.** One of the biggest mistakes that people make when starting a weight management program is failure to incorporate an exercise or strength-training program.

ACTION PRINCIPLE

Positive Attitude

A positive mental attitude comes from having a balanced life plan reinforced by daily commitment to self-improvement and service. With each day, you are closer to your goals of staying younger and living longer. You know who you are and where you are going. You know that longevity is within your reach if you follow instructions on a daily basis. You know you can do it, because you have done it before, and you are going to do it again, one day at a time. You feel the enlivening power of having control over your own future. You expect better things to happen in life. With a positive attitude, the world is a better place.

CHAPTER NINE

EAT FOR LONGEVITY

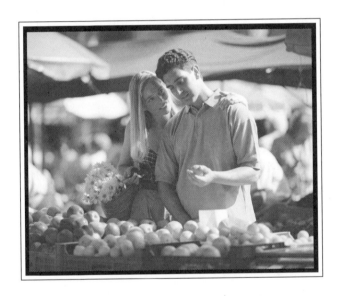

"Eat your vegetables."

Your Mother

ANTI-AGING NUTRITION

N ext to the air you breathe, food entails the largest volume and the second most frequent contact your body makes with the environment.

Anti-aging diet is not a "diet" in the sense that its objective is weight loss. An anti-aging diet is actually a lifestyle of dietary habits and an eating plan that will improve your longevity. It is, therefore, not a weight reduction diet per se, although it has weight reducing effects. To enjoy success with the anti-aging diet, you must have a thorough understanding of what it is and why it is so.

How Much Food Do You Need?

The average American consumes two to three pounds of food per day. That's 600 pounds of food per year and close to 20 tons of food over a lifetime. Knowing the right amount of food to eat is as important as knowing the right kinds to eat.

From an anti-aging perspective, most leading scientists and researchers agree that food can be used as a "drug" to defer aging. This involves the re-orientation of your thinking so that you treat food with the same respect you treat a drug. That is, take only what you need and take it with care.

As your body matures and ages, your basal metabolic rate decreases. In other words, your body's idle speed slows down. The same amount of food intake during old age is more likely to be converted into fat than protein. If you eat the same amount of food as when you were young, you will end up with fat accumulating in the familiar places such as the belly and hips. As you age, your calorie intake should be restricted to minimizing the accumulation of fat, yet be sufficient to provide enough nutrients for your body to function optimally.

Calorie Restriction (CR)

Fortunately, there is a magic elixir that can turn back the hands of time to improve the quality of life as you age. It is known as calorie restriction (CR). If you understand the consequence of over-indulgence in food is the production of excessive oxidation, an increase in fat storage, an excessive insulin load and sugar imbalance, it is easy to understand that the reverse – restricting calorie intake – has the opposite and rejuvenating effect.

For the past 60 years, **calorie restriction has been the only proven method known to reverse the aging process.** In many controlled laboratory animal studies, restricting calorie intake has resulted in test animals living a longer and more functional life with less chronic diseases. Studies over a long period of time have tried to find out why Okinawans from Japan have more than four times the centenarians per 100,000 of the population than any other section of the Japanese population. From the dietary perspective, the Okinawans eat three times more vegetables, two times as much fish, and one-third fewer calories than the standard Japanese diet. It will take many more years of scientific research to fully understand the mechanism of how calorie restriction works within your body. However, there is no doubt that it works. Do you have the time to wait, or is it smarter to follow the restrictions now, given the overwhelming amount of data and research already in place?

Benefits of Calorie Restriction

The physiological benefits of calorie restriction are many, including:

- **Increase in maximum life span**
- **Increase in learning ability (sharper mind)**
- **Increase in neurotransmitter receptors (clearer mind)**
- **Decrease in fat accumulation (better body contour)**
- **Decrease in insulin level (better sugar control)**
- **Decrease in cancer (less oxidative damage)**
- **Decrease in heart disease (less stress on the cardiovascular system)**
- **Decrease in loss of bone mass (less osteoporosis)**

How Does Calorie Restriction Work?

Calorie restriction works in three different ways.

As food intake decreases, metabolism goes down. Free radical formation as by-products of the metabolic cycle decreases. Fewer free radicals means less cellular damage and a lower likelihood of cancer and other free radical-linked diseases.

Calorie restriction causes an increase in protective enzymes such as superoxide dismutase and glutathione peroxidase, both of which oppose free radicals. The production of certain hormones such as melatonin, which has antioxidant functions, is also increased.

Calorie restriction, if properly carried out by eating more frequent, smaller meals rather than a few big meals, reduces insulin secretion and stabilizes blood sugar levels.

TOP 10 ANTI-AGING FOODS

1. Fermented Soy products such as miso and tempeh prevent cancer through isoflavones.
2. Broccoli – from the cabbage family prevents cancer through sulforaphane.
3. Peppers – red, yellow, green, or orange – increases health through capsicum.
4. Blueberries – enhances vision through anthocyanosides.
5. Tomatoes – prevents cancer through antioxidant lycopenes.
6. Garlic and Onions – enhance immune system through allium.
7. Ginger – gingerol, chemically similar to aspirin, prevents strokes.
8. Grapes – acts as anti-oxidants through flavonoids.
9. Cauliflower – prevent cancer through sulforaphane.
10. Oat Bran – soluble fiber that helps to reduce cholesterol.

Ideal Body Weight

Do you need to be on a calorie-restriction program? The answer depends largely on your current body weight and composition.

Let us take a closer look at how you can determine if you would benefit from the program. First, some basic understanding of terminology is required.

There are two kinds of weight measurement commonly used to determine if you are overweight or underweight:

1. Ideal body weight; and
2. Target anti-aging weight.

The ideal body weight is a statistical average that assumes that you are an average American in your mid-20s. If you have a special build or medical condition, the ideal body weight may not be applicable to you.

Target Anti-Aging Weight

Target anti-aging weight is the weight you want to achieve to obtain maximum longevity benefits. There is no hard and fast rule on what this should be at this stage. **From many studies where calorie restrictions of 30% to 40% were carried out in laboratory animals, longevity commonly increased by up to 100%. Most researchers in the anti-aging field find a 5% to 10% reduction from the ideal body weight a prudent and conservative approach to longevity.**

TOP 10 SUGARY FOOD BASED ON GLYCEMIC INDEX

1. Glucose — 100
2. Baked potato — 98
3. Puffed and white rice — 95
4. Corn Flakes — 80
5. Honey — 75
6. Whole grain bread — 72
7. White bread — 69
8. Raisin — 64
9. Beets — 64
10. Banana — 62

Calculating Your Ideal Body Weight and Targeting Anti-Aging Weight

If you are a female of medium frame, your ideal body weight is equal to 100 pounds plus 5 pounds for each inch above five feet. If you are five feet five inches tall, for example, your ideal body weight is 125 pounds.

To calculate your target anti-aging weight, subtract 5% to 10% from this ideal weight. Continuing with the above example, your target anti-aging weight is 104 to 110 pounds.

If you are a male of medium frame size, your ideal body weight is equal to 106 pounds plus 6 pounds for each inch you are above five feet. If you are five feet 10 inches tall, for example, your ideal body weight is 166 pounds.

To calculate your target anti-aging weight, subtract 5% to 10% from the ideal weight. Continuing with the above example, your target anti-aging weight is 157 to 149 pounds.

Add 3% to 5% to the weight if you have a big frame and likewise subtract 3% to 5% if you have a small frame.

One of the main goals, therefore, of an anti-aging diet is to achieve and/or to maintain as close as possible the target anti-aging weight so that maximum longevity is reached.

ANTI-AGING DIET

The anti-aging diet is a cuisine that is rich in fruits, vegetables, grains, omega-3 fatty acids and low in saturated fat. This diet helps to reduce the risk of heart disease, and is definitely beneficial for cancer prevention. It consists of fresh and whole foods. It is a diet high in fiber, antioxidants and other important nutrients. It is about sharing meals with family and friends, making every meal a healthy celebration. It is low in glycemic index and keeps your insulin level in check.

Let us look at the characteristics and principles of the anti-aging diet.

1. **An abundance of food from plant sources, including fruits and vegetables, beans, nuts and seeds. These foods from plant sources form the core of the anti-aging diet. Underground vegetables such as potatoes, yams and carrots are to be taken sparingly due to their high sugar content.** A diet based on this pattern is likely to be sufficient in all essential nutrients necessary to maintain health. Put food from plant rather than animal sources in the center of your plate.

2. In the anti-aging diet, using organic fruits and vegetables locally grown or gathered, seasonally fresh, is ideally consumed raw or minimally processed. That means lots of salads, as well as lightly cooked vegetables. Heavy cooking destroys enzymes required for proper digestion.

3. One of the key goals in anti-aging is to maintain a stable sugar level in the blood. Food that is quickly converted into sugar once inside the body are called high glycemic food. These should be avoided. **High glycemic foods include certain grains and vegetables such as rice, wheat, corn, potatoes and carrots.** If taken, wholegrains, whole wheat pasta, oats, or stone ground whole wheat bread or brown rice rather than food made with white refined flour, puffy processed sugar-coated cereals, or white rice, should be considered. These whole foods provide plenty of dietary fiber, antioxidants and other micronutrients that are destroyed by heat and removed by the refining process. Fruit juices have high glycemic indexes and should be avoided because of their high sugar content. Take whole fruits instead of fruit juice as they contain fiber to slow down the release of sugar, making whole fruit a lower glycemic index food.

4. **Sugar is kept to a minimum.** Special care is taken to minimize intake of sugar hidden in processed foods under names such as honey, glucose, sucrose, maltose, dextrose, high fructose corn syrup, malt syrup, as well as sugar. Sugar provides calories and calories only — no nutrients to speak of at all, which is why it is called an "empty-calorie" food. Sugar is empty of any vitamins or minerals, or phytochemicals.

FREQUENT ANTI-AGING QUESTION

Q: What is the best beverage to take for anti-aging?

Each of us takes about 180 gallons of liquids per year:

* Water   – 50 gallons
* Coffee   – 35 gallons
* Soft Drinks – 35 gallons
* Milk   – 25 gallons
* Beer   – 22 gallons
* Juices   – 8 gallons
* Tea   – 7 gallons
* Liquor/wines – 4 gallons

From an anti-aging perspective, nothing beats pure filtered water. Water is required for every cellular function in the body. Water helps detoxify and cleanse your body by helping it to remove toxins that accumulate in the cells; it is required for gaining muscle mass and burning fat; drinking water helps to hydrate the skin and helps lubricate your joints.

Your body requires at least 8 to 9 glasses of water every day. For optimal anti-aging health and insurance against premature aging, you should be drinking 12 glasses of pure filtered water throughout the day.

10 THINGS TO EAT TO PREVENT FLU

1. For Lunch — **Hot Tomato Soup**. Tomatoes contain lycopenes that act as antioxidants to help white blood cells resist free radicals.
2. For Dinner — **Garlic**. Numerous research have shown the anti-bacterial benefits of garlic. Take two to four cloves per day, or a good garlic supplement (12,000 ppm Allicin).
3. For Snack — **Natural unsweetened Yogurt**. Contains live cultures of healthy bacteria which lower the chance of coughing, colds, and wheezing, according to one study of 60 people at the University of California at Davis. (Yogurt is a dairy product that can cause allergy. The recommended intake is one to two times a week.)
4. During prolong workout — A **sports drink** to enhance immune response as advised by to a study published in the *International Journal of Sports Nutrition*.
5. At your desk — **Brazil nuts** which contain 100 mcg of selenium, a strong antioxidant that also helps prevent infections. Moderate your consumption (five nuts a day) as it is also high in fat.
6. At Dinner — low fat (25%) and not no fat (10%) diet enhance immune response while keeping cholesterol low.
7. At breakfast and dinner — a well rounded high potency **multi-vitamin and antioxidant supplement**.
8. At afternoon tea — **Celery and Carrot sticks** that contain vitamin C and other antioxidants instead of sandwiches that raise blood sugar levels.
9. Bedtime snack — **Try to avoid** if possible. Sugar reduces our immunity and defense system and increases control of the pro-aging hormone. A glass of warm water is best to hydrate the cells.
10. Upon awakening — drink at least two glasses of water (8 ounces each) to rid the toxins that have remained in your body over the evening. Water will clear your system and prevent stasis of toxins.

1. **Dairy products are avoided.** They are usually in the form of cheese and yogurt, principally coming from a variety of animals such as goat, sheep, water buffalo, cow and camel. Not only do they cause many allergies in the body, they are also high in fat and animal protein that accelerates the aging process.

2. Weekly consumption of moderate amounts of deep water fish and free-range poultry.

3. Red meat is only taken a few times per month (consumption should be limited to a total maximum of 12 to 16 ounces per month, preferably lean versions). It is high in saturated fat and is difficult to digest.

4. Whole Fresh fruit is the typical daily dessert. Sweets and saturated fat desserts should not be consumed more than once a week. Total fat should be less than 25% to 30% of energy with saturated fat not more than 7% to 8% of energy (calories).

5. Olive oil and canola oil, the major sources of fat in the anti-aging diet, are high in mono-unsaturated fat and to be encouraged.

ANTI-AGING FOOD PYRAMID

Based on the above anti-aging principles the Anti-Aging Food Choice Pyramid was created. It consists of 50% to 55% complex carbohydrates of low glycemic nature (such as barley and oats, and whole grain cereals.) High glycemic grains such as refined wheat, white rice, and corn as well as underground vegetables such as potatoes and carrots should be avoided). This diet

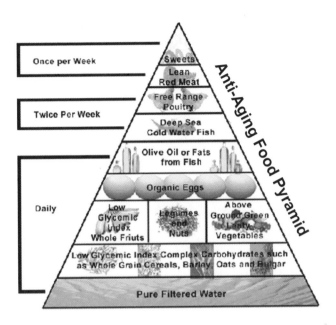

comprises 20% to 25% protein preferably from plant and fish sources, 25% to 30% fat, and 5% sweets, candies, and dessert.

This is a sharp contrast to the typical North American diet in which 46% of the calories are from carbohydrates, 11% from protein, and 43% from fat.

Imagine a pyramid with multiple layers, each layer getting much narrower as it gets closer to the top. The broad base layer of the pyramid starts with 10 to 15 glasses of pure filtered water a day. Complement that with daily intake of low glycemic index carbohydrates such as barley and oats, whole grain pastas, cereals, low glycemic whole fruits, legumes, above ground vegetables and eggs on a daily basis. Try to avoid white breads, white rice, corn and pasta as they are high in glycemic index. Use olive oil or canola oil as a source of fat in cooking.

In the middle of the pyramid and to be taken two to three times a week are cold-water deep-sea fish, such as salmon, tuna and free-range chicken. These will supply plenty of protein.

Lean red meats and desserts such as ice cream should form no more than 5% of the diet and to be taken only once a week. These are at the top of the pyramid.

FREQUENT ANTI-AGING QUESTION

Q: Are there any food that speed up the aging process?

Saturated fat, excessive protein, fried foods, and sugar from your diet create free radicals in your liver, and also make you feel sluggish. Increased free radicals in the body will increase oxidative damages, which can lead to degenerative diseases and cancer.

ANTI-AGING DIETARY TIPS

Staying youthful is equal to staying healthy. They go hand in hand; and staying healthy is governed, to a large degree, by your daily habits of eating. If your eating habits have become just habits with little thought put into them, your diet will probably be unbalanced in nutrients and calories. Keep in mind that quality of life starts at the level of nourishment for each of your cells.

The following dietary guidelines will help you to incorporate sound nutritional habits into your daily life. These are simple tips that are especially useful if your focus has not been on a balanced diet before:

1. **Be aware of the amount of calories you need to maintain your ideal weight; 5% to 10% below ideal body weight is a good target to shoot for.**

2. **Eat like a king at breakfast, a prince at lunch, and a pauper at dinner.** Breakfast is the most important meal as it provides important nutrients you need to start the day. In addition, the calories from breakfast give you energy in the morning, and you have all day to burn them off. Dinner should be the lightest meal of the day because there is less time for the meal to be digested and the calories to be burned off.

3. You should chew your food at least 20 times before swallowing. **One way to restrict calorie intake without feeling deprived is to eat slowly, savoring each mouthful.** You must resist the hectic pace of modern living, which discourages you from taking enough time to eat in a healthful way. To eat slowly means you will no longer gulp your food, washing each mouthful down with fluid. Instead, you will chew each mouthful thoroughly so that it is easier to swallow without additional fluids.

    There are at least three advantages to doing this. Firstly, the proper amount of chewing prepares the food more adequately for the stomach and digestion. Humans do not produce enzymes that destroy plant cell walls, but those cell walls have to be broken so that the vitamins, minerals, phytochemicals, antioxidants, etc, that they enclose can escape and be made available to us. Cooking helps to disintegrate those walls somewhat and chewing helps to complete the job by mechanically breaking the walls. Without adequate mastication, much of the valuable nutrients in plant food passes right through you, remaining locked in their cells, so you do not get as much nutrients as you think you are getting.

The second advantage of chewing well is that your stomach will not have to work so hard or so long to get the food to the right consistency for digestion.

The third reason has to do with caloric restriction. When you chew more, you feel more satisfied with the same amount of food. You also take longer to eat, allowing the appestat in your brain, which takes about 20 minutes to kick in, to say, "Hey, you've eaten enough. Call it quits." People who gulp their food have finished their meal before their appestat has had enough time to work, and often eat more than they need without feeling satisfied.

4. **Reduce overall fat and sugar intake as they provide only empty calories,** calories without other beneficial nutrients, resulting in a *calorie*-dense diet. The anti-aging diet, on the other hand, is a *nutrient*-dense diet, meaning every calorie comes with other nutrients as well. That is one reason that fruits are recommended as the major source of sweetness in your diet, since the calories from fruits are accompanied by vitamins, minerals, antioxidants, phytochemicals and various kinds of fibers, which are essential for anti-aging and for keeping the body youthful. Further, the body prefers to use carbohydrates for energy, so that calories consumed as fat get stored as fat.

5. **Whole food are more nutritious than refined food**. That means using whole grains like 100% percent whole wheat bread and brown rice rather than white bread or rice; oats, Shreddies™ and whole grain cereals rather than puffed rice, or sugared flakes, and puffs. It means using the whole fruit rather than just the juice, though a little juice has its place. **All refining processes remove important nutrients.** In addition, the refining process removes the fiber, which, although not a nutrient, has many anti-aging effects.

    The richest source of antioxidants in grain is found in the germ, which is removed in the refining process. The highest percentage of minerals and vitamins in the grain is found in the germ and the bran layer, which are removed in the refining process. But what about enrichment? **If you were robbed of $100, would you consider yourself "enriched" because the robber decided to return $40 to you?** In the enrichment process, only a small proportion of both amount and type of nutrients that were removed in the refining process, are replaced. Besides providing more nutrition, whole foods also help you maintain a steady blood sugar level.

6. **Eat a variety from the plant food**. Eat from each group — fruits, vegetables, grains, legumes, nuts and seeds. Within the fruit group, eat a variety. Within the vegetable group, eat vegetables of all different colors; eat leafy vegetables, vegetables with stems, flowers, roots, and those that surround their seeds (like squash and tomatoes, which are technically fruit) For grains, there are more than just wheat and corn. There are oats, rye, barley, triticale, and others. There are also hundreds of legumes such as black eye peas, split peas, green peas, navy, kidney, lima and garbanzo beans, and of course, soybeans and lentils. By doing this, you will be less

---

FREQUENT ANTI-AGING QUESTION

Q: So many doctors recommend a high protein, low carbohydrate diet. Are these diets harmful to my body?

A high protein diet can potentially strain the kidneys and acidify the body. Every day, amino acids that are not needed for building the body have their nitrogen removed, and are converted to carbohydrates for energy. The extra nitrogen must be processed and excreted by the kidneys. A sufficient intake of water (10 to 12 glasses per day) is necessary to keep the kidneys functioning properly if you are on a high protein diet.

---

likely to miss out on any necessary vitamins, minerals or phytochemicals.

7.   **You do not need vast amounts of protein in your diet. Experiment with meat substitutes or non-animal protein foods such as tofu and legumes.** Eat more deep water fish, organically fed chicken and very little red meat. Vegetable proteins are perfectly adequate. The amino acids that are low in grains are supplied in legumes, or nuts and vice versa, which is another reason to eat a variety of foods. Grains and legumes do not have a be eaten at the same meal. Any time during the same day is sufficient. All proteins, from whatever source, are broken down and remade into your own unique proteins. Further, plant proteins are free of cholesterol, and saturated fats and the toxins that are found in animal protein sources.

8. **Include organically grown foods in your diet.** Chemically laden food is a burden to the body. Even small amounts of toxin accumulate and eventually wear down the body organs and cause premature aging.

9. **Drink at least eight glasses of pure filtered water every day in order to remain healthy.** Water helps you to get rid of the toxins and unwanted waste materials from your body. It also keeps you hydrated, helping to prevent premature aging of the skin and joints. Adequate amounts of water are necessary to prevent body temperatures from rising too high when exercising, or in hot weather.

10. **Allergy prone individuals should avoid milk and other dairy products** because dairy products are mucous-forming and have a high potential for allergic reactions. Further, as you age, you do not have the enzymes necessary to break down the milk sugars. Therefore, you may experience gas, bloating, nausea, diarrhea and often gall bladder distress.

11. **Install a good water filter, not only for the kitchen sink but also for the tub and shower as well.** Most of the nation's water supply is contaminated by agricultural run-off, manufacturing waste, fluoride, chlorine and other chemicals and chemical by-products. A good water filter system should include multi-stages to remove bacteria as small as 1 micron or less. Furthermore the water should be slightly alkalinized to reach a pH of 7.4 to 7.6. Ultra violet disinfection is normally not necessary if you have a ceramic or carbon block filter. The better filtration devices also have built in magnet and microlization apparatus to reduce the size of water cluster and enhance water absorption into the cell for optimum health contains caffeine because caffeine causes unnecessary stimulation of the nervous system.

12. **Avoid fried foods.** They normally contain the worse kind of fat (trans-fat) for your body. Steam, broil or stir-fry whenever possible.

13. Avoid drinking coffee, black tea, red tea, green tea, cola type sodas or **anything else that contains caffeine because caffeine causes unnecessary stimulation of the nervous system.**

14. **The best way to lose excess weight is to eliminate saturated fat, excessive protein and sugar from your diet.** These foods create free radicals in your liver and also make you feel sluggish.

15. **Eat six small meals per day, rather than the traditional three square meals.** This way, you will maintain a balance in your blood sugar and the level of nutrients in your body throughout the day.

DINING OUT TIPS

If you eat out only occasionally, you may be able to order whatever you desire; but if you eat out regularly, choosing foods high in calories, fat and cholesterol can harm your health. By simply staying away from some of the items you typically order, you can eat more healthily, and still eat out. Here are some simple tips to help you stay on your anti-aging diet track when you dine out:

1. **Ask for small or half-size portions at sit-down restaurants**, or consider splitting an entrée with a friend or bringing half the meal home or having an appetizer as your entrée.

2. Be familiar with portion sizes:
   - 4 ounces of meat or fish looks like a deck of cards or a computer mouse;
   - 1 cup of cooked vegetables looks like a baseball;
   - 1 ounce of cheese looks like a wine cork; and
   - 1 teaspoon of butter looks like 2/3 of a standard pat.

3. Ask that gravy, butter, rich sauces, and salad dressings be served on the side so you can control the amount you eat.

4. **Ask to substitute a salad or baked potato for chips, fries or other extras.**

5. **When ordering pizza, choose vegetable toppings** like green pepper, onions, and mushrooms instead of meat toppings or extra cheese.

6. **At the salad bar, fill-up on vegetables**. Limit intake of food like bacon and cheese, and prepared salads like potato or macaroni salad. Go easy on the salad dressings – and choose low-calorie dressing or oil and vinegar when it's offered, or use a squeeze of lemon juice.

7. At fast-food restaurants, **choose small sizes of food** and drinks. Order salads and grilled chicken or fish sandwiches with no sauce.

8. Many restaurants now offer heart-healthy entrees or smaller portions for people who are watching their weight or their cholesterol levels. When the menu does not spell out smarter food choices, try to avoid certain selections: pasta swimming in heavy cream, deep-fried side dishes, rich desserts.

9. Order broth-based soups such as minestrone, vegetable or chicken noodle rather than cream soups. When ordering a sandwich, ask for whole grain bread or whole wheat bread. For lower fat meats, the best choices are turkey or chicken breast and lean roast beef. Try a vegetarian sandwich with grilled Portobello mushroom, peppers, zucchini or eggplant slices. A slice of reduced fat or part-skimmed cheese is also delicious cold or melted in a sandwich. Add lots of veggies to make your sandwich complete. Lettuce is always a good addition, but use darker versions for more nutrition. Tomatoes, cucumbers, onions, peppers, and sprouts also add flavor, crunch, fiber, and nutrients.

FREQUENT ANTI-AGING QUESTION

Q: Why is eating six small meals is better than three big meals?

Eating six small meals per day, rather than the traditional three square meals, will help your body maintain a balance in your blood sugar, and prevent diabetes and prolong life.

You are what you breathe, eat, and digest. Proper nutrition is critical for optimum cellular function. The **Anti-Aging Food Pyramid** is designed to do this through your daily meals. It is specially designed to combat age-related degenerative diseases such as diabetes, cardiovascular disease, high cholesterol, hypertension, and cancer by normalizing sugar, reducing oxidative stress, and improving the immune function. In short, **it keeps you younger and live longer.**

CHAPTER TEN

EAT YOUR WAY OUT
OF DEGENERATIVE DISEASES

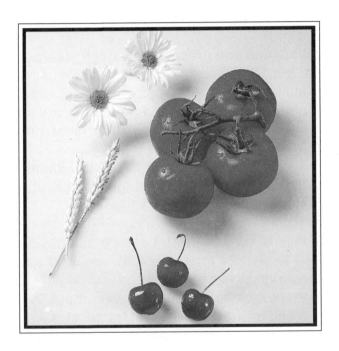

*"Treat food as a drug
and you will live longer."*
Dr Michael Lam, MD

THERAPEUTIC NUTRITION

Only a century ago, cancer, atherosclerosis, hypertension, and diabetes were virtually unknown.

At that time, people relied more on whole raw foods, unrefined and generally in their original form fresh from the farm. The introduction of refined sugar (eg soda pop) in the late 1800s, then canning in the early 1900s, followed by processed food in the 1940s changed this picture drastically.

Food when canned and processed is not the same as that in its original form. Commercialization produces a longer shelf life that translated into higher profit for food manufacturers. **Natural vitamins, minerals, enzymes, and co-factors are stripped in the process, and the chemical structure of nutrients is changed.** What goes in is different from what comes out of the processing plant. **Processed food is not the same as "raw" food that occurs in nature, that are high in fiber, antioxidants, and nutrients.**

Over 2 pounds of food is taken by each one of us everyday. This equates to over **20 tons** over a lifetime. Is it possible that what you feed yourself has no bearing on your health? The normal degenerative process of the body takes about **20 years to progress from initial insult to disease state.** Continued excessive intake of processed foods and sugar leads to a variety of age-related degenerative diseases starting at about the age of 40, 20 years after the body hit peak performance at age 20.

The use of nutrition and dietary adjustments as a tool to prevent and treat diseases is **as old as human history itself.**

Since the advent of modern medicine over the last hundred years, society has rushed to this new-found method of "quick fixes" that is supposed to cure diseases painlessly simply by taking pills. It is quite amazing how quickly the public has abandoned what has been the norm for 5,000 years.

After 100 years of modern medicine, the number of people suffering from chronic age-related degenerative diseases such as hypertension, heart diseases, and diabetes continues to skyrocket despite the best medical effort. Modern medicine has utterly failed to cure chronic degenerative diseases.

Why? Let us consider the following.

1. High Blood Pressure

MYTH
Too much fluid in the blood vessel causes high blood pressure.

TRADITIONAL TREATMENT
Removal of excess fluid through the use of diuretics. This is often the first line of treatment. This is augmented with vasodilators. Amazingly, most people believe this distorted explanation without question.

DISCUSSION
More than 43 million Americans have high blood pressure (hypertension), but **less than one third of them have achieved targeted levels of blood pressure with medication.** Even among the 23.4 million who take anti-hypertensive medication, **only 42.9% of these patients actually get their blood pressure down to acceptable levels.**

FACT
One of the primary causes of high blood pressure is the loss of fluids. The less fluids in the body, the more the blood vessels constricts in an auto regulatory attempt to increase the pressure

so that valuable blood flow and oxygen is delivered to the brain and various parts of the body. **Diuretics increase dehydration.** They make you lose more water, and promote a vicious cycle of increasing blood vessel constriction which in turn cause higher blood pressure In other words, **high blood pressure is often a symptom of dehydration.**

NATURAL SOLUTION

Drink more water! By adding more water to the body system, the heart would not be so desperate to hang onto both sodium and water. Increased blood volume also makes the blood more diluted. With increased blood flow, the negative feedback system kicks in to dilate the blood vessels and open them up wider, resulting in the lowering of blood pressure. Such a simple method consistently **lowers blood pressure on a long-term basis.**

2. Cancer

FACT

The majority of cancer is **genetically linked or are related to lifestyle factors.** The real cause is still unknown for most types of cancer.

TRADITIONAL TREATMENT

The standard treatment of cancer involves **surgery, chemotherapy, and radiotherapy.**

DISCUSSION

Cancer is perhaps the most humbling part of traditional medicine. Most researchers acknowledge that we are still in our infancy as far as understanding how cells become cancerous. Most researchers, including Nobel Prize winner Sir MacFarlane Burnet, feel that in the normal body hundreds of cancer cells appear every day. It is a normal part of the oxidative process and cellular function. Cancer cells are routinely destroyed by the body's internal immune system. Often when this system fails, cancer arises.

Cancer is a general condition that localizes, rather than being a local condition which generalizes. A tumor is often a symptom of a failing immune system.

The majority of cancers are not symptomatic. In fact, most are found during autopsy. It can be said that our current laboratory test is not sensitive enough to detect minute cancer cells. Equally, it should be stressed that most cancer cells do not cause any symptoms. In fact, 30 to 40 times as many cases of thyroid, pancreatic, and prostate cancer are found in autopsies than ever. According to a study published in top British medical journal, the *Lancet* (13 February 1993), early screening is good, but the aggressive nature of traditional medical approach often leads to unnecessary treatment. A 1992 study was reported in the *Journal of the American Medical Association*: out of 223 patients, it was concluded that no treatment at all for prostate cancer was actually better than any standard chemotherapy, radiation or surgical procedure.

FACT
More people are dying of cancer now per capita than ever before, and nothing is slowing the increase. Not early detection, not better screenings, not radiation, surgery, nor chemotherapy. Sometimes, toxic and lethal chemo therapeutic drugs are used. Cancer cells are stimulated and they strive to survive any way they can by increasing their growth as they struggle for survival. This normal process of adaptation buys some time, and often those who have had chemotherapy normally experience temporary remission. The tumor ultimately returns, and does so with vengeance. **Our body's immune system is built to combat cancer cells when its growth compromises our organ function.** Our immune system can hold many problems in check, as long as it is not compromised by powerful insults. **Maintaining a strong immune system is the key to anti-aging, as most cancers become detected after the age of 40.**

Strengthen your immune system. The best way to prevent or defer cancer formation is by following the anti-aging diet and taking extra antioxidants that enhance the immune system.

3. Peptic Ulcer Disease (PUD)

MYTH

PUD is caused by an **increase in acid secretion in the gastric system**. The cause of this is still unknown.

TRADITIONAL TREATMENT

Millions of people around the world take **antacids or drugs to block acid secretion**.

DISCUSSION

In his book, *The Body's Many Cries for Water,* Dr Batmanghelidj reported his successful treatment of 3,000 peptic ulcer patients using water alone and nothing else. He explains how **ulcer pain is really a thirst-warning signal.** It makes perfect sense: in situations where the intestine is too dehydrated to adequately refresh its mucus lining every time after the acidic products of digestion have passed by, the lining will become irritated. Long-term irritation leads to erosion of the gastric lining, leading to pain and peptic ulcer. The intestine is not protected from digestive acid like the stomach is. **Antacids will only relief the pain temporarily and cover up the problem. Rehydrating the gastro-intestinal tract will enable the intestine to form adequate mucous lining, thus reducing acid irritation.**

FACT

PUD may well be the first symptom of chronic dehydration and not a disease by itself.

Drink plenty of water, especially when you have the gastric pain. Take at least ten glasses of pure filtered water a day as a minimum for optimum anti-aging health, and more if heavy physical activities are undertaken.

4. High Cholesterol

High blood cholesterol is mainly caused by **high cholesterol intake in the diet**.

Suppress cholesterol production in the liver by administration of **cholesterol lowering statin drugs.**

While statin drugs are effective in lowering the total cholesterol and amount of LDL cholesterol, they have **serious side effects**. For years, the public was led to believe that the wonders of statin drugs was not only in lowering cholesterol but also in possessing other health benefits as well. Millions of statin prescriptions are written yearly in the United States alone. In August 2001, however, German Pharmaceutical giant Bayer AG withdrew the cholesterol-lowering statin drug Baycol from the market because it was linked to 31 deaths. Moreover, deaths occurred at the manufacturer's recommended initial dose (0.4 mg/day) as well as at the highest dose (0.8 mg/day). The majority of deaths occurred in elderly patients and more often in women.

High total serum cholesterol and LDL cholesterol are significant risk factors of cardiovascular disease. Fourteen million Americans have heart disease and more than 2,600 die daily from heart attacks in the United States alone. Fifteen percent of adults in their late 30s to 40s are afflicted with cardiovascular disease, about 50% of 55 to 64-year-olds, and 65% of those in the next decade.

Developed countries have shown a **decrease in dietary fat and cholesterol consumption in recent years.** This is largely the result of on-going massive public health campaign advocating a low fat, high carbohydrate diet as ideal to bring down· blood cholesterol level to prevent atherosclerosis. Despite this effort, **the number of people with elevated blood cholesterol continues to increase**. Obviously, there are other causative factors that have not been addressed. In America alone, over 40 million prescriptions are written yearly for cholesterol lowering medications.

Studies have shown that **a diet high in cholesterol will not lead to high blood cholesterol if the subject is healthy**. Blood cholesterol level only increases by 3 mg/dl after ingestion of one egg each day for a continuous period of six weeks (one egg contains about 230 mg cholesterol) in repeated studies. Clearly, **dietary cholesterol is not the main culprit.**

High sugar intake is linked to an increased risk of heart disease. Simple sugars are the primary source of high triglycerides, a type of blood fat, and very low-density lipoproteins (VLDL), which are an independent risk factor for atherosclerosis. **Sugar lowers good HDL cholesterol and raises bad LDL cholesterol and blood pressure levels.** It is estimated that a high sugar intake may account for as many as 150,000 premature deaths from heart disease in the US each year.

Sugar increases triglyceride storage and cellular oxidative damage. This assaults the vascular wall, leading to micro-leakages in the endothelial wall of blood vessels. The body tries to patch up the leakage by increasing production of cholesterol and lipoprotein (a) production from the liver. Sugar is, therefore, a significant contributory factor of oxidative stress. Simple logic dictates that reduction of sugar intake will reduce oxidative stress. This in turn will reduce cholesterol production from the liver.

FACT
Elevated cholesterol is primarily symptom of oxidative stress and not a disease.

NATURAL SOLUTION
The real cause of elevated cholesterol level is oxidative damage from excessive free radical damage caused by excessive metabolism of oxygen and sugar. Humans lack the endogenous capacity to produce vitamin C, a natural antioxidant. Instead, the body produces cholesterol as a surrogate repair nutrient. If you understand this concept, it is easy to appreciate that high cholesterol and a host of other age-related diseases such as atherosclerosis are nothing more than a series of symptoms reflective of the body's response to imbalanced oxygen and sugar metabolism. **To normalize cholesterol level permanently, proper control of your oxygen load (through reduction of oxidative stress by taking antioxidants) and sugar load (by avoiding foods that are high in sugar and concentrating on low glycemic index food) is the first and most important step, in addition to exercise.**

5.   Atherosclerosis

MYTH
Atherosclerosis is **caused by high dietary fat and cholesterol,** lack of exercise and high stress.

TRADITIONAL TREATMENT
Low fat diet, exercise, and reduction stress.

DISCUSSION
Some researchers believe that cardiovascular disease is primarily caused by **chronic deficiencies of vitamins and other essential**

nutrients with defined biochemical properties, such as coenzymes, cellular energy carriers, and antioxidants. Chronic depletion of these essential nutrients in endothelial and vascular smooth muscle cells impair their ability to function properly. Take the effects of vitamin C (ascorbic acid) deficiency as an example. **Humans, other primates, and guinea pigs do not produce ascorbate endogenously.** Guinea-pigs fed a diet low in ascorbate, an amount equivalent to the usual human intake, rapidly developed atherosclerotic plaques, similar to those found in humans. When large amounts of supplementary ascorbate were given to these guinea pigs, there was a regression in plaque formation. Humans must get vitamin C from external sources. Deficiency of vitamin C leads to a disease called scurvy, the symptoms of which causes the reduced ability of the body to make collagen, an essential component of wound healing, bones and joints, and blood vessels. **Chronic ascorbate deficiency leads to impairment in the structure of the blood vessel walls and tiny lesions in its inner wall. These changes are the hallmarks of early atherosclerosis.**

In a landmark study published in the *Journal of Applied Nutrition* (1996, 48:3), researchers showed that **coronary artery disease could be effectively prevented and treated by natural means**. In patients with early coronary calcification, progression was halted. In individual cases with small-calcified deposits, optimum nutritional supplement intervention led to the complete disappearance of the deposits.

FACT
Coronary artery disease is a symptom of chronic vitamin C deficiency.

SOLUTION
Take optimum doses of **vitamin C (ascorbic acid), ascorbic palmitate, amino acids L-proline and L-lysine**.

CHAPTER ELEVEN

STRESS MANAGEMENT

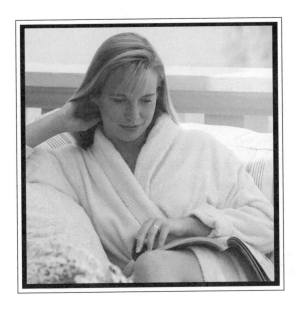

*"The greatest discovery of my generation
is that man can alter his life simply
by altering his attitude of mind."*

James Truslow Adams

S tress is a killer. Researchers estimate that stress contributes to the majority of our major illnesses, including cancer, cardiovascular and metabolic diseases, skin disorders and infectious ailments of all kinds. Stress is also a common denominator in many psychological difficulties such as depression and anxiety.

DIFFERENT KINDS OF STRESS

While stress is an unavoidable part of life, it can result from many different factors, both physical and psychological. Pressures and deadlines at work, problems with loved ones, financial obligations and the simple acts of getting ready for holidays are some obvious sources of stress for many people. Less obvious sources include everyday encounters with crowds, noise, traffic, temperature changes, new job, birth or adoption of a child. Overwork, the lack of sleep, as well as physical illnesses are some common physical factors that increase stress in our body. Some people are able to deal with stress in a creative way and minimize distress when it occurs. Some people even thrive on stress and for these, they create their stress without knowing it. Most people, however, are negatively influenced by it.

Stress can cause fatigue, chronic headache, irritability, change in appetite, memory loss, low self-esteem, withdrawal, high blood pressure, shallow breathing, nervous twitches, low sexual drive and a variety of gastro-intestinal disorders. The writing on the wall is clear — stress is a killer!

> ## Top 10 Mindset To Become 100
>
> 1. **Believe** that you want to live to 100.
> 2. **Find meaning** in life.
> 3. Be an **optimist**.
> 4. **Take risk and be creative**.
> 5. Be a good neighbor — **stay in touch**.
> 6. **Stimulate your brain** by learning and building memory.
> 7. Keep **family** structure strong.
> 8. **Work with stress** — do not take life so seriously.
> 9. **Be attractive**.
> 10. **Give**, not only to your friends and family, but also to strangers your wealth of knowledge gained over the years.

How Does Stress Shorten Our Life Span?

Almost all body organs and functions react to stress. The pituitary gland increases its production of adrenocorticotropic hormone (ACTH), which is a precursor to the release of two hormones called cortisone and cortisol. These two hormones have the effect of inhibiting the functions of disease fighting white blood cells and suppressing the immune response. This complex of physical changes is called the "fight or flight response." While most of our stresses in modern day society are not a result of physical threat, the body responses are the same, whether the threat is physical or psychological.

The increase in production of these hormones is responsible for most of the symptoms associated with stress. Increase in the production of these hormones causes the body to step up its metabolism of protein, fat, and carbohydrate to quickly produce energy for the body to use during its "fight or flight" state. This response causes the body to excrete amino acid, potassium and a variety of minerals like magnesium that are vital to the body's defense mode. Furthermore, the body is not able to absorb digestive nutrients well when under stress. The intestinal tract is often affected. In severe cases, bleeding may result due to the high level secretion of gastric acid during times of stress.

Many disorders that arise from stress can also result from nutritional deficiency, especially deficiency of the B-complex vitamins, which are very important for the proper functioning of the nervous system.

Goal of Stress Reduction

While stress is part and parcel of everyday life, it should be remembered that it is not stress that is detrimental to your health and decreasing longevity. All human life needs stress to a certain degree to survive well and be productive. It is your reaction to the daily stresses of life and your body's reactions to it that is responsible for how long you live.

STRESS MANAGEMENT

So how are we supposed to deal with stress? Most of us have a healthy "personal escape" that we use to deal with daily stresses. They can classified into three broad categories:

1. Mental activities such as reading, listening to music, playing chess.
2. Physical activities such as gardening, shopping, fishing, walking.
3. Functional activities such as massage, aromatherapy, spa.

FREQUENT ANTI-AGING QUESTION

Q: How do I cope with stress while driving? I often feel tense and get very angry and upset when someone beeps a horn or cuts me off.

Road rage is a very common source of stress for those who live in metropolitan areas. First, look at the source of your frustration. Are you exhausted and frustrated by long hours at work, or is the stress and tension of balancing work and family driving you crazy? Next, try to alternate your routes to create variation. Last of all, try simple breathing exercises while driving, or listen to your favorite music.

It is no use getting upset at other drivers. It is like a domino effect where your frustration will cause the other driver to become more aggressive (no matter who is at fault). The result can be tragic. Instead, take a deep breath and let it slide. Your health and safety is not worth another driver's inconsiderate behavior.

Use these activities to help take you away from the stresses of daily life. Put on those headphones and be transported to another place. Go for a jog and simply concentrate on your form and technique. Get a massage and let all your worries slip away.

Many people enjoy all three types of activities. The important thing to remember is that you should find something that helps you to relax and use it as your personal escape whenever you find yourself needing to unwind.

Stress Reduction Tips

There is no one magic bullet for stress reduction. Everyone's likes and dislikes are different. The following are some common stress reduction techniques that work.

Physical Exercise

Physical activity can clear your mind and keep stress under control. Some people like to run or walk by themselves while others prefer various team sports. **Any type of exercise is good, and it is even better if it is regular.** Stress is built up through a period of time and gradual reduction is the best way to reduce stress. Next time you feel stressed out, go to the gym or simply take a walk. This is a good first step of any stress reduction program.

Learn to Relax

Relaxation is more difficult for some people to attain than others. Some are born relaxed while others are more tense. This is particularly true of the type A hyperactive individual, who thrives on a high degree of stress and chaos in his or her life.

ACTION PRINCIPLE

Stay Disciplined

In the battle of life, you will take plenty of punches. Some come from the left without warning and you have to take it. Some come from the front, but you are too slow to see it. You can see some coming, but you are too confident that it will not hit you. These punches hurt, but they make you smarter and more disciplined. The discipline helps you to stay focused so that you can avoid new punches. The older you get, the more disciplined you become because you do not want to take too many more punches.

Discipline to follow the five pillars of anti-aging discussed in this book will help you dodge cardiovascular cancer, stroke, and many other age related diseases. You win a fight by striking at the right time and dodging punches.

Here is a simple but effective way to learn how to relax. It involves learning to tighten and relax the body's major muscle groups, one at a time, being aware of each sensation. Start at your feet and work your way up to your head. Tense your muscle and count to ten, concentrating on the tension. Let the muscle go lax and breathe deeply, enjoying the sensation of each release. Performing this simple progressive and relaxing exercise while you are lying down in a quiet room can work wonders.

Gain Sufficient Sleep

Many people cannot sleep with stress. **A restful night is a key ingredient to help many people deal with the daily stresses of life.** If you have a lot of stress, getting a good night's sleep is an important thing to do. Some people, however, have a tendency to escape stress by resorting to excessive sleeping during stressful situations. If you are one of these people, then you should not sleep more than the usual.

Meditation

For centuries, meditation has helped thousands of people to relax and handle stress. Meditation does not necessarily have a spiritual or religious connotation. There are a wide variety of ways to meditate, some of which concentrate on a religious belief while others have no specific beliefs associated. One can meditate on such words as "calm" or "relax."

Like anything else, meditation has short-term benefits as well as long-term effects. Long-term effects are usually the most pronounced, but only after consistent performance on a daily basis.

Deep Breathing

This is perhaps the most simple and easiest stress reduction technique. Deep breathing is also convenient to do, whether you are at home, at work or in a car. Breathe with your mouth closed, hold your breath for 3 seconds, and then exhale slowly through your mouth, with your tongue placed at the top of your teeth. Do this four to five times, or until the tension has passed.

FREQUENT ANTI-AGING QUESTION

Q: Does what I eat make a difference when I am stressed out?

Studies show that certain foods tend to be stress reducing, like complex carbohydrates – pasta, potatoes – that are more slowly absorbed. Do not skip meals when you are stressed. Your body becomes stressed when it is deprived of nutrients for long periods of time. In terms of what you eat, stay away from the usual villains like sugary snacks. Watch the coffee and the hidden stimulants in things like medicines, colas, and some bottled waters containing caffeine.

Create A Stress-Free Home Environment

Keep the noise level down as noise contributes to stress. Create a meditation room where you can be in a quiet environment with natural sounds (such as a babbling brook) in the background, without the noise of TV and cars. Use as much natural lighting in your home as possible, as unnatural fluorescent lighting can be particularly aggravating.

Aromatherapy

This is the art of using highly concentrated distilled herbal essences, called essential oils. Add 10 to 12 drops or more of these oils to a warm bath and relax in the tub. Or simply dab a couple of drops of oil on a tissue or handkerchief and inhale the aroma during the day.

Professional Counseling

If you cannot handle the stress in your life, consider outside help. Professional counselors are available to help enlighten your thought processes. It is often beneficial to talk to someone who can offer an objective response and give us a different view of how we should look at the world.

Qigong

Qigong is a Chinese form of meditation plus yoga-type exercises, that require years to master. Many millions of people around the world practice this quiet form of yoga-cum-meditation art that originated in China. There are many qigong clubs around the country, so you may want to join one to get started.

CHAPTER TWELVE

ANTI-AGING STRATEGIES

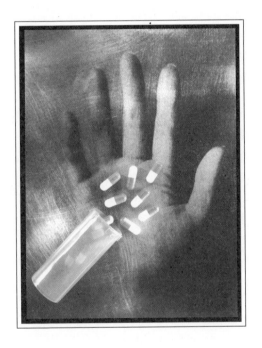

*"A beautiful lady is an accident of nature.
A beautiful old lady is a work of art."*
Louis Nizer

ANTI-AGING STRATEGIES

This chapter summarizes over **100 specific anti-aging strategies** that took over a decade to compile. Every strategy is based on scientific research backed by years of clinical experience. **They are grouped according to the five pillars of anti-aging medicine:**

1. diet;
2. exercise;
3. hormonal enhancement;
4. nutritional supplement; and
5. stress reduction.

Those new to this should read this daily for the **first 21 days.** A thorough understanding of each strategy is critical before embarking on the journey. Do not adapt any strategy unless you know the reason and the consequences. Certain strategies are uniquely suited for you while others may not be. Do what makes sense for you and you alone, as each body is different.

Do not attempt any quick transformation. Most transformations fail because of too high an expectation in too limited a time. **Go slow, one step at a time.** Your body has gone through a lifetime of damage. Recovery and rejuvenation is a process that works best when it is slow and steady. The path to anti-aging is a marathon and not a sprint.

While there are no absolutes in life, it should be remembered that the law of averages still apply in anti-aging.

In most cases:
1. people who smoke do not get lung cancer;
2. people who forget their seat belts do not die in traffic accidents;
3. people who have unprotected sex do not contract AIDS;
4. people who go on diets do not become anorexic; and
5. people who are sun worshippers do not get skin cancer.

Nevertheless, **those who follow these anti-aging strategies will generally feel:**

1. **younger;**
2. **healthier;**
3. **lighter; and**
4. **more energetic.**

Complete fulfilment of these strategies requires significant lifestyle adjustments for most. No one is expected to adopt 100 percent of the recommended strategies all the time. A successful execution of the anti-aging strategies takes generally from **1 to 3 years**. Consider yourself doing well if you can follow 25% of the strategies within 90 to 180 days, 50 % of the strategies within 1 to 2 years, and 75% of the strategies within 2 to 3 years. The body is a miraculous machine. It is very forgiving and does rejuvenate, starting at the cellular level.

Expect to see **some results after 30 to 90 days** after you have selected those strategies you wish to embark on first. Select easy strategies first and slowly work your way into more difficult ones. Rome was not built in one day. Concentrate on learning, listening, and loving your body and it will take care of you.

Our life expectancy has already doubled in the past century, from 43 to 76 for those in developed countries. This is largely due to the discovery of antibiotics and successful execution of anti-aging strategies such as these. They have worked in the past and will continue to work in the future. Longevity is 70 percent is determined by lifestyle and 30 percent related to genetics. What you can do is to work on the lifestyle related 70 percent today, since therapeutic modalities for the other genetically related 30 percent is still years away from reality.

1. DIET

VEGETABLES
DO

- **Do eat more organic vegetables** (they taste better and has three times more nutrients). The stronger the color, the higher the nutritional level.
- **Do eat kale, spinach, green and red cabbage, broccoli, red and green leaf lettuce, romaine lettuce, cauliflower, zucchini, Chinese cabbage, bok choy, and cucumbers**. These are all **vegetables grown above the ground** and are high in antioxidants, minerals, vitamins, and fiber.
- **Do rinse your vegetables well** to kill germs and spin it down well to prolong shelf life. Wash all fresh fruits and vegetables with cool tap water immediately before eating. Do not use soap on them. Scrub firm produce such as melons and cucumbers with a clean produce brush. Cut away any bruised or damaged areas before eating.
- **Do squeeze the air out** of the bag if you intent to store vegetables. Fresh produce should be refrigerated within two hours of peeling or cutting.

DO NOT

- **Do not eat iceberg lettuce**. It is mostly water, low in fiber and nutrition.
- **Do not eat underground vegetables** such as carrots and potatoes that are high in sugar (high glycemic index) that can trigger diabetes. Mashed potato is acceptable due to the addition of fat and milk *during* the cooking process.

GRAINS AND SUGAR

DO NOT

- **Do not take refined sugar**. Adding sugar to food is common and socially acceptable. It reduces your immune system function. Sugar in your food goes rapidly to your blood. When there is excess sugar in your blood, your liver may use it to make more triglycerides. This contributes to higher blood serum triglycerides, cholesterol, promoting obesity due to higher fatty acid storage around organs and in subcutaneous tissue folds. Over consumption of sugar is the leading cause of diabetes, heart attack, and cancer.
- **Do not take high glycemic index grains such as rice, wheat, and corn.** They cause a sugar spike increase in the blood and contribute to diabetes, obesity, and heart disease. If high glycemic food is combined with protein and fat in a meal, the glycemic index is lowered, resulting in a slower release of sugar into the bloodstream.
- **Do not take corn or corn related products** such as popcorn (hard to digest and of minimal nutritive value) and chips (high in fat). Corn is not a vegetable but a grain.
- **Do not take artificial sugar** such as aspartame and artificial flavoring such as MSG. Both contain chemicals that produce well-documented damage to your body.

PROTEIN
DO

* **Do get protein from beans and legumes** — make sure beans are well soaked for 48 to 72 hours prior to cooking, to help digestion and ensure that they are cooked thoroughly in a crock-pot for at least eight hours to break down harmful toxins.
* **Do get protein from raw seeds** such as sunflower, pumpkin, sesame, and flax. The consumption amount should be limited because these are also high in fat.
* **Do get protein in limited amount from raw nuts** such as Brazil nuts, cashews, and almonds. The consumption amount should be limited because these are also high in fat.
* **Do get protein from organic eggs** that come from organically fed free-range chicken. Egg white is one of the best and cheapest sources of protein.
* **Do get protein from cold and deep water fish** such as salmon and tuna. Avoid fish from coastal waters that are easily contaminated with toxins such as mercury.
* **Do get protein from lean meat from animal**. Lean meat from **grass fed cattle,** not commercially raised grain fed cattle, is preferred.

DO NOT

* **Do not get protein from foods derived from scavengers,** such as **pork, ham, most bacon, shellfish, shrimps, lobsters, crabs, and clams.** They are often contaminated.
* **Do not get protein from processed, cured, smoked, or dried meats,** such as bacon, sausage, ham, hot dogs, or luncheon meats.
* **Do not get protein from peanuts**. Its is high in fat and often allergenic.

- **Do not get protein from soy unless it is fermented such as tempeh or miso.**
- **Do not get protein from diary products, including milk and cheese.** Pasteurization is the problem as it destroys the nutrients and changes the structure of many enzymes. Cheese in small amounts is acceptable. Yogurt from pasteurized milk should also be avoided.

FRUITS
DO

- **Do eat whole fruits that are high in fiber and low in sugar**, such as blueberries and apples, but only in moderate amounts.
- **Do peel all fruits and vegetables**, unless they are to be thoroughly cooked. Wash your hands afterwards. If you cannot peel them, soak them for 15 minutes in a solution made by adding one teaspoon of 3% hydrogen peroxide to two quarts of water, and then rinsing thoroughly with filtered water.

DO NOT

- **Do not eat bananas or watermelon** that are high in sugars and low in fiber.

FAT AND CHOLESTEROL
DO

- **Do eat plenty of deep and cold water fish** like tuna and salmon that contain a plentiful supply of omega-3 essential fatty acid.
- **Do take flex seed**, raw sunflower and pumpkin seeds.
- **Do take butter.** Even though a diary product, the amount of milk protein casein is small.

DO NOT

- **Do not be afraid of eggs as a source of cholesterol**. Choose organic eggs from organically fed chicken. Cholesterol is needed for a healthy body. Moderate consumption of one to two eggs per day does not significantly increase your blood cholesterol level if you are in good health. The best way to cook eggs is to hard-boil them. Organic eggs contain a 1:1 omega 6 to omega 3 ratio. Commercial eggs, on the other hand, contain up to 15:1 omega-6 to omega-3 ratio. Commercial eggs are not unhealthy due to cholesterol, but due to the excessive level of omega 6.
- **Do not eat trans-fat.** This is the worse kind of fat you can take. Trans-fat is found in margarine, doughnuts, cookies, pastries, deep-fat fried foods such as french fries, potato chips, and imitation cheeses.

FLUIDS

DO

- **Do take pure filtered water only**, preferably from the reverse osmosis process. Bottled water is the next best option. Take at least 10 to 12 glasses a day. Your body can process about one glass per hour. The excess is flushed out of the kidneys. Thirst is a sign of dehydration in its late stages. Keep a bottle of water with you whenever you are out during the day.
- **Do take fresh vegetable juice** (not fruit juice). A two-step extraction and press process is the best.
- **Do store water in a glass and not plastic container**.
- **Do drink more water when exercising.** Drink up before you work out. Take in about 16 to 20 ounces of either water or sports drink one to two hours prior to activity. This extra fluid will help offset sweat losses; any excess will be excreted as urine before you work out. Take in 5 to 12 ounces of either

water or sports drink every 15 to 20 minutes of exercise. If you work out for more than an hour, choose sports drinks.

DO NOT

- **Do not drink tap water**, as it is full of contaminants and chlorine. Stay away from drinks containing fluoride. If you have no choice, make sure that boiled tap water has been kept at a rolling boil for at least five minutes.
- **Do not drink distilled water**, unless for a short-term detoxification process because it can lead to de-mineralization with long-term use due to its acidic properties.
- **Do not drink coffee.** It is a stimulant and a diuretic. Heavy coffee drinkers should taper off slowly. One cup a day is acceptable.
- **Do not drink fruit juice**, especially those that have a high concentration of sugar. Each glass of juice can contain up to eight teaspoons of sugar. Take fiber-filled whole fruit in moderate quantity as an alternative.
- **Do not drink tea**, including red, black, and green tea. Tea is a stimulant. Green tea contains antioxidants, but fruits and vegetables are better sources. It also contains fluoride. Herb tea is acceptable as it is not really tea but a herbal infusion in a tea bag.
- **Do not take soda pop**. It is full of sugar and empty nutrition. Aluminum from the can is toxic.
- **Do not take milk** – not needed for adults, especially skimmed milk. Milk protein casein is the culprit, aside from the fact that milk is highly allergenic.
- **Do not over drink wine and alcohol**. Drinking too much wine – or any alcoholic beverage – has a definite downside. Numerous studies suggest that consuming more than two drinks a day over the long-term may raise blood pressure in

some people and increase the risk for strokes and other diseases.

What, When and How to Eat

* **Meals:** Breakfast – full (eggs and vegetable juice is best); Lunch – moderate; Dinner – small and early. Do take a walk immediately after a meal to promote circulation.
* **Calorie:** Eat to 70% fullness. Maintain a diet of 1500 to 1800 calories a day if you are sedentary to achieve a target anti-aging weight at or slightly below your ideal body weight (men: 106 pounds for first 5 feet in height plus 6 pounds for each addition inch above 5 feet; women: 100 pounds for the first 5 feet plus 5 pounds for each inch above 5 feet).
* **Dessert: Only at lunch.** Avoid before-bed snacks, particularly grains and sugars. This will raise blood sugar and inhibit sleep. A few hours later, reactive hypoglycemia may take place and you may wake up and not be able to get back to sleep. Late-night snacks high in sugar also promote the release of cortisol, an pro-aging hormone you can do without.
* **Microwave: Do not use** to heat food as it changes the molecular structure of the nutrients. High frequency electromagnetic waves that alternate in positive and negative directions are used, causing vibration of food molecules up to 2.5 billion times per second. Heat created as a result can destroy the structure of vitamins and enzymes.
* **Chew food thoroughly** (20 times each mouthful) before swallowing in order to aid digestion.
* **Do not take too much water** with your food, which can dilute the digestive enzymes.

- **Do not take genetically engineered food**. Available only since 1995, there is simply not enough information on the long-term heath effect. It is hard to conceive that there are no structural changes to the nutrients that have been genetically modified. The damage may be insidious, similar to smoking, and it may require many decades of ingestion to observe the effects. The risks are not worth taking.
- **Do not take irradiated food**. From a nutritional perspective, irradiation is like exposing food to the equivalent of up to 1 billion chest x-rays that depletes vitamins, often significantly. Especially vulnerable are vitamins A, B-complex, C, E, and beta-carotene. For instance, irradiation destroys up to 80% of the vitamin A in eggs, and about half of the thiamin in wheat flour. Essential fatty acids can be damaged, as can amino acids. Furthermore, beneficial micro-organisms are killed along with the harmful ones. Animals that ate irradiated food faced premature death, fatal internal bleeding, a rare form of cancer, stillbirths and other reproductive problems, genetic damage, organ malfunctions and nutritional deficiencies, to name a few. Scientists have little or no idea whether irradiated food is safe for human consumption.

Diet Summary: Take plenty of green leafy vegetables, moderate amounts of lean meat from grass-fed cattle, farm-raised poultry and cold-water fish as a source of protein is acceptable. Avoid grains and underground vegetables such as potatoes and carrots. Organic eggs, raw nuts, and seeds are rich sources of protein. Fat is good, especially from cold water fish that is rich in omega 3 fatty acid. Stay away from trans-fat such as french fries and cookies. Take pure filtered water only. Cook with olive oil (monounsaturated), coconut oil (already saturated), canola oil (monounsaturated and polyunsaturated) and butter. Eat a big breakfast, moderate lunch, and early and light dinner. Avoid dessert at night. Chew your food well. Eat to 70% fullness, and do not use microwave to cook your food.

2. EXERCISE

DO

- **Do be active**. A sedentary lifestyle is twice as likely to kill you as a high cholesterol level. Long-term studies have shown that those least fit were eight times more likely to die of heart or cardiovascular disease than the most fit. Physical inactivity causes osteoporosis, the loss of calcium that makes bones brittle and fracture-prone. An individual confined to bed will lose up to 4% of bone mass within a month.
- **Do strength training exercise**, especially with the large muscle groups (chest, back, and thigh) at least **three times a week, 15 minutes each** time to increase growth hormone secretion. Strength training induces the development of additional new muscle cells and more resilient tendons, ligaments, and muscles. Added strength improves neuromuscular control, which in turn protects you from injury. Strength training is especially important for the back, since lower-back pain is often caused by weakness of the abdominal and/or back muscles.
- **Do cardiovascular exercise everyday**, **30 minutes** total at 80% of maximum heart rate (maximum heart rate is equal to 220 less your age). Breaking up exercise into short bursts of activity throughout the day strengthens the heart just as well as one long workout session. You can break down the 20 minutes into two sessions of 10 minutes each. Studies show that heart disease risk was found to depend more on how many overall calories were burned. Men who burned

4,400 calories per week through exercise are nearly 40% less likely to develop heart disease than are men who use up only 1,100 calories per week. This effect holds, regardless of whether the men walked, climbed stairs, or played sports. Do not forget that golf is not an aerobic sport.

- **Do flexibility training 5 minutes before and after each exercise session** to warm up and cool down the muscles, ensure smooth joint movement, prevent accidents, and maintain good balance.

- **Do drink extra water** when you exercise to **avoid dehydration.** Sports drinks are acceptable. Check the label: your sports drink should provide about 50 to 80 calories per eight-ounce serving (this translates to 14g to 20g of carbohydrates per serving). After you finish an activity, drink two cups of fluid for every pound lost during your workout.

- **Do exercise in mid-afternoon,** which is the safest if you have no special preference. Often your body will tell you when the most comfortable time is. Follow your body rhythm for best results.

- **Do be consistent in your exercise program.** The is the secret of success.

- **Do create variety in your exercise program.** Cross-training is any fitness program that systematically incorporates a variety of activities to promote balanced fitness. Instead of just running, swimming, bicycling, aerobics classes or just any single activity, cross-training is participating in several different exercise activities.

- **Do exercise as far from traffic and pollution as you can.** You do not want to undo exercise's health benefits by exposure to carbon monoxide, ozone, oxides of sulfur and nitrogen, particulate matter, and hundreds of other toxic chemicals. Increased depth and rate of breathing during aerobic exercise magnifies the detrimental effects of polluted air.

DO NOT

- **Do not over-exercise**. The human body is not made to sustain the structural damage from a marathon. It is good for the ego but not for the body. Sustained over-exercising can cause damage at a rate faster than the body's ability to heal. This will wear you out prematurely. Not only is there no upside to excessive training but by generating more free radicals than the body is prepared to scavenge, over-training actually weakens the immune system and increases susceptibility to degenerative disease. Consistency is far more important than intensity. **Expenditure over 3,500 to 4,000 calories a week is considered excessive from an anti-aging perspective. Target to spend 2000 to 3000 calories a week from exercise.**
- **Do not make exercise too complicated**. A simple exercise program that can be done anywhere is the key.
- **Do not compare yourself with others**. Each person is unique and is at a different level of fitness.
- **Do not try to get fit by being active**. You can become more active only by becoming fit.

3. NUTRITIONAL SUPPLEMENTATION

DO

- Do take a well rounded **multiple vitamin and mineral formula** cocktail in optimum anti-aging dose to prevent oxidative stress. Different vitamins and minerals work on different parts of the cell. There is no one magic bullet. The body needs about **40 different micronutrients** for optimum function.

- **Do take additional function specific nutritional supplements** for aging conditions such as memory lost, high cholesterol, high blood sugar, heart function, immunity, and cancer prevention.
- **Do take your supplements with meals** to enhance absorption.
- **Do take your supplements everyday.**
- **Do take digestive enzymes and probiotics** to enhance gastrointestinal health. Active cultures of Lactobacillus and Acidophilus promote normal flora in the gut.
- **Do take magnesium.** Eighty percent of the adult population is deficient in magnesium even by RDA standards. Magnesium, together with vitamin C and E, is a critical anti-aging mineral because it is required in optimum mitochondrial function. 500 to 1,000 mg in divided dose is preferred. If you have diarrhea, back off and stay at the dose where no diarrhea occurs.

DO NOT

- **Do not use supplements as a substitute of good whole foods**.
- **Do not take Iron** as part of an anti-aging supplement program unless you are anaemic.
- **Do not take supplements if they smell bad.**

4. STRESS REDUCTION

DO

- **Do develop a personal stress reduction program** uniquely suited to your lifestyle and likes. Doing what is relaxing to you is the key. Do not compare with others. What works for one person may not work for another.

- **Do breath properly to reduce stresses and tensions of everyday life.** Use your diaphragm and not your chest wall.
- **Do develop a close circle of trusted friends** to share your stress.
- **Do take things in your stride.**
- **Do follow an exercise program.** It is by far the best stress reducer.

DO NOT

- **Do not avoid all stress.** Some stress is necessary for a happy life.
- **Do not overeat or oversleep** as an escape when faced with stress.
- **Do not overreact and act emotionally.** Take a break when faced with stress you cannot handle.

5. HORMONAL ENHANCEMENT

DO

- **Do strength training of large muscle groups** such as chest, back, and thigh three times a week, 15 minutes each time to enhance endogenous growth hormone release.
- **Do aerobics exercises 30 minutes each day** to enhance endogenous growth hormone release.
- **Do restrict calorie intake** by eating to 70% fullness. This has been shown to promote growth hormone release endogenously.
- **Do consider progesterone replacement and natural hormonal replacement therapy** as an alternative to traditional treatments of menopausal symptoms.

- **Do consider nutritional supplementation** such as vitamin E and evening primrose oil to modulate hormonal cycle for women. For men, the prevention of Benign Prostate Hypertrophy and delaying the onset of andropause through vitamins, herbs, and minerals are important.
- **Do take amino acids** like glutamine that acts as a secretagogue to enhance endogenous release of growth hormone.

6. MISCELLANEOUS STRATEGIES

DO

- **Do use a shower filter** to avoid chlorine exposure from tap water during showers.
- **Do keep the kitchen counter clean.** Cutting boards, dishes, utensils, and counter tops should be washed with hot, soapy water and sanitized after coming in contact with fresh produce or raw meat, poultry, or seafood. Sanitize after use with a solution of one teaspoon of chlorine bleach in one quart of water. Leave your dishwashing sponge very dry and without any residue of organic material. Clean the sponge after you wash the dishes, and keep it away from the cutting board.
- **Do watch out for toxic molds.** Mold toxins (mycotoxins) may suppress the immune system and cause cancer. Refrigerators are a haven for mold, which loves to grow on bruised fruits and vegetables. If a hard food that is uncooked becomes moldy, cut and discard the moldy part and at least one inch of the food in each direction from the site of mold. ("Hard" foods include apples, broccoli, carrots, cauliflower, and hard cheese in chunks, garlic cloves, onions, pears, potatoes, squash and turnips.) If a soft food, juice or cooked leftover becomes moldy, throw it all away; do not attempt to salvage any of it.

- **Do** listen to your body. It will tell you far in advance what is wrong. Every body is unique and different. Accept the fact that it is far more important to listen to your body in addition to listening to your doctor.
- **Do expose your body to at least 30 minutes of direct or indirect** sunlight **per day**. Small amounts of daily sunshine on our skin and in our eyes are critical to good health. Apply sunscreen as needed.
- **Do avoid electromagnetic fields** such as cellular phones, electric blankets, and a home near electrical plants. Avoid wearing metals, including jewelry.
- **Do take drugs only as a last resort**. All drugs have side effects. Avoid antacids and acid lowering drugs. The body's first line of defense against intestinal infection is the acid produced by a healthy stomach. Stomach acid kills most of the bacteria and parasites that are swallowed along with meals. Strong suppression of stomach acid increases the risk of intestinal infection. It is also important to avoid unnecessary antibiotics. The second line of defense against intestinal infection is the normal intestinal bacteria, especially Lactobacilli residing in the small intestine. Antibiotics decimate Lactobacilli. In so doing, they increase the risk of subsequent intestinal infections.
- **Do see your doctor for routine** medical checkups and to rid yourself of any toxic metals like mercury, lead, and arsenic in your body.
- **Do have daily bowel movement** that should be effortless and odorless. Stool should not sink to the bottom of the bowl.
- **Do inspect your urine.** It should be clear to very light yellow color. Dark color could mean infection and dehydration, unless you are on B vitamins.

- **Do** sleep in total darkness without night-light to maximize melatonin production. When light hits the eyes, it disrupts the circadian rhythm of the pineal gland and the production of melatonin and serotonin.
- **Do replace all silver amalgam dental fillings** (actually contain 50% mercury). Avoid ceramic and porcelain crowns as they have metal in them. Use composites. Avoid toothpaste with fluoride.
- **Do follow a** detoxification program, including regular fasting, skin brushing, colon cleansing, sauna, and steam baths.
- **Do pray in time of sickness.** Numerous studies have confirmed the power of prayer in healing with statistical significance. Clinical studies have reported that heart patients who receive prayer have 50% to 100% fewer side effects.

DO NOT

- **Do not initiate too fast a lifestyle change** that can act as a stressor to your body, especially if lifelong habits have been well established. Give yourself one to two years for transition to an anti-aging lifestyle, slowly and one step at a time.
- **Do not stop smoking immediately** if you have been smoking for a long time, but do stop sugar intake. Studies have shown that 65 mg of vitamin C is needed to counteract the free radical and oxidative stress damage of one cigarette.
- **Do not use antiperspirants.** Generally full of aluminum, which is a toxic substance and has been linked to Alzheimer's disease.
- **Do not use aluminium, teflon coated, and stainless steel cookwares.** Enamel coated metal or glassware is best as they are inert and will not add toxic metal to the food.

CHAPTER THIRTEEN

MEASURING SUCCESS

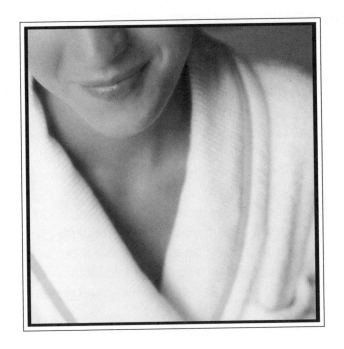

"Numbers don't lie."

Anonymous

INTRODUCTION

S uccess in the anti-aging program comes from knowing that you have done your best to attain the knowledge and have taken action to do what is best for your body. This internal feeling of well being and self-actualization is the ultimate success reward of the anti-aging program.

The number of marathons you can run, or your percent body fat therefore does not strictly measure success in anti-aging. These are but a few gauge to help you realize your goal and serves as a marker to let you know if you are on track or not in your anti-aging program.

The fact that you are doing the 5 components of anti-aging: Proper diet, exercise, taking supplementation, making an effort to reduce the daily stresses of life, and taking appropriate hormone replacement therapy, is already a success. There are no failures.

Some basic baseline measurements before and during your anti-aging program serves as objective tool to measure your progress. If you have a camera, don't be afraid to take pictures of yourself. This will serve as the best motivation factor for years to come as you look back and vow to never be what you have been.

Here are some easy to do test that you can perform every 3 months to gauge your progress. Record them on your diary and be proud of yourself for taking the effort which is what counts.

MEASURING GENERAL BODY CONTOUR AND COMPOSITION

A. WEIGHT

Anti-Aging body weight is equal to your ideal body weight less 5% (up to 10% is even better)

Try the following formula:
For ladies: (105 lbs + 5 lbs for every inch of height above 5 feet) x 0.95
For men: (106 lbs + 6 lbs for every inch of height above 5 feet) x 0.95

Goal: Maintain weight at anti-aging body weight consistently

B. BODY FAT ANALYSIS

Percent Body Fat

Take the following measurements:
1. Hip at the greatest circumference area
2. Thigh at the widest part of the upper thigh
3. Wrist just above the bony protuberance toward the hand
4. Calf at the widest part, about midway between the knee and the ankle
5. Forearm at the widest part, about midway between the wrist and the elbow

Body Fat for:
Women under 30 = hip + (0.8 x thigh) - (2 x calf) - wrist
Women over 30 = hip + thigh - (2 x calf) - wrist
Men 30 and under =waist + (1/2 hip) - (3 x forearm) - wrist
Men over 30 = waist + (1/2 hip) - (2.7 x forearm) - wrist

Accuracy:

While the total body immersion test is the most accurate, it is cumbersome and impractical. This simple method has a accuracy level to +/- 2%.

If you are very fit, numbers from this test may be 3-5% above the total body immersion test because they have cleaned out their intramuscular fat.

If you are skinny but not fit, the result from this test may be 3-5% lower than the immersion test because skinny people have more than the usual amount of fat inside their muscle.

The national average men is 22%, and the average women is 32%
Healthy for men is under 15
Obese for men is over 30

Best anti-aging range for men is 10-15
Healthy for women is under 22
Obese for women is over 33
Best anti-aging range for women is 15-22

How many pounds of fat do you have?
Pounds of fat = total weight x % body fat
the amount of fat you should have = total body weight in pounds
X % * (*15% for men, 22% for women)
the amount of fat you need to loose / gain = difference

How many pounds of lean body mass do you have?
Pounds of lean body mass do you have = total weight in pounds - (total weight x % body fat)

The amount of lean body mass you should have = total body weight - pounds of body fat

The amount of lean body mass you should have = total body weight in pounds x %*   (* = 85% for men and 78% for women)

C. MEASURING YOUR FLEXIBILITY

Test: sit and reach test

Procedure:

a. You need a measuring sick or tape, and some adhesive tape.
b. Lay the measuring stick on the floor and place a 12 inch piece of adhesive tape long ways across the 15 inch mark of the ruler.
c. Without your shoes on, sit on the floor with your heels at the tape line, about 12 inches apart, and the zero mark of the ruler towards your body.
d. Keep your knees straight and hands together as you reach forward.
e. Stretch as far as possible, holding the furthest position for 3 seconds. Don't bounce or allow one hand to reach farther than the other.
f. Record the effort.

Flexibility Test Results

	MEN	WOMEN
Excellent	> 19.5	> 22.5
Very good	17.25-19.5	19.5- 22.5
Good	15.5 - 17.25	18.25- 19.5
Average	13.75 - 15.5	16.75- 18.25
Below average	11.5 - 13.75	15.25- 16.75
Poor	9.0- 11.5	12.5- 15.25
Very poor	< 9	< 12.5

D. MEASURING YOUR CARDIOVASCULAR FUNCTION

1 mile fitness walking test:

How: walk as fast as you can for 1 mile, either on a track or flat surface (treadmill is OK).

Immediately after completion of the mile, take a pulse count and note both completion time in minutes and heart rate per minute. Measure how long it takes you to cover 1 mile in a comfortable aerobic pace. You should be running at a comfortable pace that would enable you to carry out a conversation without feeling out of breath.

AEROBIC PACE RANGE (MIN/MILE)	AGE 20-44	AGE 45 AND OVER	ACCEPTABLE FOR ANTI-AGING
6	Excellent	Excellent	
7-8	Very good	Excellent	
9-10	Above average	Very good	Yes
11-13	Average	Above average	Yes
14-17	Below average	Average	Yes
18-20	Poor	Below average	
>21	Very poor	Poor	

E. MEASURING YOUR STRENGTH CAPACITY

a. Vital Statistics

- Chest (inhale) at the nipple line
- Chest (exhale) at the nipple line
- Upper arm (relax) at maximal biceps

- Upper arm (contract) with biceps relaxed
- Waist at the top of the hip bone (iliac crest)
- Hip at the biggest area of your glutes (buttock)
- Thigh at the largest part
- Calf at the largest part

b. Measuring your Maximum Strength

Test: One-Rep Max Test
One-rep max (1 RM) represents the heaviest amount of weight you can properly lift for only one repetition.

Procedure:
Once you have warmed up, take up to 3 attempts to determine your correct 1 RM weight, allowing yourself 5 minutes of rest between each attempt. Always use a spotter. However, he or she should not help with the weights unless you absolutely cannot lit it any further.

Bench Press: _____   Leg Press: _____

10 MARKERS OF GOOD HEALTH

The following are 10 markers that will help to direct you towards optimum health. If you follow the anti-aging life-style, you should be able to achieve the following relatively easy after 3-6 months on the program.

1. Anti-aging body weight = ideal body weight less 5-10%
2. Systolic blood pressure under 120 regardless of age
3. Percent body fat under 15% for male and under 22% for female
4. Able to Bench Press at least 50% of your weight
5. Fast walk or jog at comfortable pace for a mile in under 15 minutes
6. Serum DHEA level at high end of normal for age
7. Serum albumin level towards high end of normal
8. Serum Cholesterol level 180-200, with HDL > 45 and LDL > 130
9. Serum ferritin level within normal limits
10. Serum homocysteine level within normal limits
11. Serum Lipoprotein (a) within normal limits

Anti-aging Program Flow Sheet (do every 3 months)

DATE	GOAL		
BASIC STATISTICS			
Ideal Body Weight			
Current Weight (CW)			
Anti-Aging Target Weight (AATW)	IBW - 5%		
Weight you need to loose (in pounds)	CW-ATW		
% body fat currently (% BF)	M<15, F<22		
Pounds of body fat currently (BF)	CW x %BF		
Anti-Aging Pounds of fat to have (AABF)	ATW x0.15 for men (0.22 for female)		
Pounds of Fat to loose	BF- AABF		
Pounds of lean body mass currently (LBM)	CW - BF		
Pounds of lean body mass you should have (AALBM)	ATW X 0.85 for men (and 0.78 for ladies)		
Pounds of lean body mass you need to gain	AALBM-LBM		
FLEXIBILITY STATUS			
Flexibility Test	M: 15-17 F: 18-20		
CARDIOVASCULAR STATUS			
1 mile fitness test	11-13 min		
BODY CONTOUR STATUS			
Chest (inhale) at the nipple line			
Chest (exhale) at the nipple line			
Upper arm (relax) at maximal biceps			
Upper arm (contract) with biceps relaxed			
Waist at the top of the hip bone (iliac crest)			
Hip at the biggest area of your glutes (buttock)			
Thigh at the largest part			
Calf at the largest part			
STRENGTH STATUS			
Bench Press (1 RM)	>50% of weight		
Leg Press (1 RM)	>50% of weight		
VITAL SIGNS			
Systolic Blood Pressure	<120 regardless of age		
Resting Pulse Rate per min	< 80 regardless of age		
BLOOD TEST			
Serum Cholesterol	180-200 mg/dl		
Serum HDL level	>45 mg/dl		
Serum Albumin Level	>48 gm/l		
Serum DHEA level	at top end of range for age		
Serum Ferritin level	within range		
Serum Homocysteine level	under 8 umol/l		

Women's Optimum Daily Allowance

VERY IMPORTANT

Vitamin A/Beta Carotene (Antioxidant) – total of 25,000 IU (300% RDA) with no more than 5,000 IU in Vitamin A Palmitate and the rest in natural mixed beta carotene. More than 100 studies have shown that people with high levels of beta carotene in their diet have half the chance of developing cancer and heart attack.

Vitamin C (Antioxidant) – 1000 mg (2000% RDA) in the form of ascorbic acid (not necessary to spend more money on other forms unless you have a sensitive stomach or taking more than 2,000 to 3,000 mg per day). A study of Americans show that intake of 300 mg of vitamin C per day adds six years to a man's life and two years to a woman's life. Cardiovascular disease decreased by 40%. Take this in split dosages as it is secreted within a few hours. No toxicity has been reported on long-term intake of up to 20,000 mg a day. **It is important to incorporate Ascobyl Palmitate (the fat soluble form of vitamin C) , L-proline, and L-lysine as well. The three work synergistically to rebuild damaged blood vessels and prevent atherosclerosis.**

Vitamin E (Antioxidant) – 400 IU (1333% RDA) to 800 IU in the form of water dispersible d-alpha tocopherol (the natural form). This amount has been shown in repeated researches to be the optimum dose for anti-aging and cancer prevention. The risk of not taking vitamin E is statistically equivalent to the risk of smoking. A large scale Harvard study of 87,000 nurses showed that those taking more than 250 IU a day for two years have 41% lower incidence of major heart disease. To take the equivalent of 400 IU in food would require two quarts of corn oil or 28 cups of peanuts a day. **Many in the fore front of anti-aging research are now recommending up to 800 IU a day, especially for women in peri- or post-menopausal period.**

Selenium (Antioxidant) – 200 mcg (285 % RDA) in amino acid complex form to enhance absorption. Selenium is a strong antioxidant and the level in our body falls with age. People with decreased levels of selenium are associated with higher incidence of heart disease, cancer, and arthritis.

Magnesium (Antioxidant) – 500 to 1000 mg (125% to 250% RDA). Less than 25% of Americans meet the low RDA standard. A 2,000 kcal diet is needed if no supplement is taken. This is critical for proper heart function, to normalize arrhythmias, and helps to reduce blood pressure. Requirement is higher if your intake of sugar and fat is high in your diet. The calcium to magnesium ratio should be between 1:1 to 1:2.

Vitamin B9 (folic acid) – 800 mcg (200% RDA) a non-toxic nutrient that protects our chromosome from DNA damage and cancer. A Harvard study of 16,000 women and 9,500 men showed that those getting the most folic acid had the lowest incidence of getting pre-cancerous polyps in the colon. Folic acid also helps with depression. No noticeable side effects at up to 10,000 mcg.

Vitamin B12 – 100 mcg to 1,000 mcg (1,666% to 16,666% RDA). Over 24% of people over 60 years old and over 40% of people over 80 years old are deficient due to decreased absorption with age. Deficiency also causes symptoms similar to Alzheimer's disease. A must take for those over 50 years old as cheap and added insurance. Non-toxic at 1,000 mcg daily for many years or up to 100,000 mcg in a single dose.

Chromium – 200 mcg (166% RDA) in chelated form for better absorption. Very little is contained in food and as a result, 90% of all Americans are deficient in the RDA of this trace element which is critical to normalize blood sugar. An Israeli research shows that daily intake of 200 mcg of chromium improves insulin resistance in Type II Diabetes by up to 50 % in weeks.

Zinc – 30 to 50 mg (200% RDA) in chelated form for better absorption. Thirty-three percent of healthy Americans over age 50 have zinc deficiency and do not know it. The percentage increases to 90% for those older. You need a daily calorie intake of 2,400 kcal to get just the RDA. Zinc is critical for proper thymus gland and immune system function. Research has shown that daily intake of 30 mg of zinc stimulates the immune system with dramatic improvements after 6 months in those with zinc deficiency.

Calcium – 500 mg (50% RDA) in the form of calcium carbonate. Calcium is important. In addition to keeping our bones healthy, calcium also fights cancer. Calcium carbonate contains 40% calcium, compare to others such as calcium glutamate that contains 9% elemental calcium. Do not take more than 500 mg at a time for best absorption. Calcium citrate is better absorbed, but only contains 11% calcium. Calcium should be balanced with magnesium at 1:1 or 1:2 ratio.

Citrus Bioflavonoids – 100 mg. Potent antioxidants derived from plants that have metal binding (chelating) properties. Commonly found in grape seed.

Omega-3 Fatty Acid – Eating 8 ounces of fish a week is all you need to do. If not, then take 1,000 mg from fish oil to contain 360 mg EPA and 240 mg DHA. Most people taking fish oil have a tendency to develop a fishy "burp". Over 60 research studies have shown that a variety of ailments from arthritis to heart disease can benefit from fish oil (not cod liver oil which contains high dose of vitamins A and D, which is toxic); 400 IU of Vitamin E should be taken simultaneously to potentiate the effect of fish oil.

Garlic – 500 mg in concentrated form, equivalent to 1250 mg garlic bulk or half a clove of fresh garlic. Garlic has been used by healers for over 5,000 years. Numerous studies have shown that garlic decreases triglyceride level by decreasing fat absorption. It also supports healthy blood pressure. Garlic's major compounds, allicin, have been found to possess powerful actions that help the body boost its immune power. A natural herb that is non-toxic.

Evening Primrose Oil – 500 mg to 1,000 mg (standardized to 9% GLA). An essential fatty acid. Strong anti-inflammatory properties and useful for arthritis, PMS, and skin conditions. Most researches use 3,000 to 6,000 mg a day. EPO is especially good for balancing the hormonal system.

Digestive Enzymes contain lipase, cellulase, protease and amylase.

Avoid **Iron unless You are Anemic.**

IMPORTANT

Vitamin B1 (thiamine) – 100 mg (6,666% RDA) – critical for mental function and nerve cell growth. Non toxic and water soluble.

Vitamin B2 (riboflavin) – 50 mg (2,940% RDA) – required for cell growth and release of energy, formation of red blood cell, and synthesis of antibodies.

Vitamin B3 (niacin) – 190 mg (950% RDA) in the form of niacin and niacinamide-stabilizes cell membranes, ensures proper circulation and maintains healthy skin. Aids in the function of the nervous system and helps to reduce cholesterol.

Vitamin B5 (panthothenic acid) – 400 mg (4,000% RDA) – a non toxic nutrient needed to breakdown fat to covert into energy. An anti-stress vitamin.

Vitamin B7 (biotin) – 300 mcg (100% RDA) – essential for protein, fat and carbohydrate metabolism. Helps in the utilization of other B complex vitamins.

Iodine 150 mcg (100% RDA) – important for the proper maintenance of the thyroid function.

Maganese 20 mg (1,000% RDA) – trace mineral essential for protein and fat metabolism.

Molybdenum 50 mcg (66% RDA) – essential trace mineral for nitrogen metabolism.

Potassium 99 mg – critical for normal cardiac rhythm.

Boron 2 mg – enhances healthy bone and brain function and alertness.

Silicon 2.4 mg – needed in formation of collagen and connective tissues.

Vanadium 25 mcg – essential in formation of bone and teeth.

L-Lysine 200 mg – an essential amino acid for proper growth in children and protein synthesis in adults.

Choline 200 mg – responsible for proper neurotransmitter function, lecithin formation, liver function, and gall bladder regulation.

Inositol 100 mg – vital for hair growth and prevention of arteries from hardening.

PABA (para-aminobenzoic acid) – basic constituent of many B complex vitamins and antioxidants. Helps protect against sunburn and skin cancer.

Men's Optimum Daily Allowance

VERY IMPORTANT

Vitamin A/Beta Carotene (Antioxidant) – 25,000 IU (300% RDA) with no more than 5,000 IU in Vitamin A Palmitate and the rest in natural mixed beta carotene. You will not get overdosed or suffer toxic effects. More than 100 studies have shown that people with high levels of beta carotene in their diet have half the chance of developing cancer and heart attack.

Vitamin C (Antioxidant) – 1000 mg (2,000% RDA) in the form of ascorbic acid (not necessary to spend more money on other forms unless you have a sensitive stomach or are taking more than 2,000 to 3,000 mg per day). A study of Americans show that intake of 300 mg of vitamin C per day adds six years to a man's life and two years to a woman's life. Cardiovascular disease decreased by 40%. Take this in split dosages as it is secreted within a few hours. No toxicity has been reported on long-term intake of up to 20,000 mg a day. **It is important to incorporate Ascobyl Palmitate (the fat soluble form of vitamin C), L-proline, and L-lysine as well. The three work synergistically to rebuild damaged blood vessels and prevent atherosclerosis.**

Vitamin E (Antioxidant) – 300 to 400 IU (1,333% RDA) in the form of water dispersible d-alpha tocopherol (the natural form). This amount has been shown in repeated researches to be the optimum dose for anti-aging and cancer prevention. The risk in taking sugar and fat and not taking vitamin E is statistically equivalent to the risk of smoking. A large scale Harvard study of 87,000 nurses showed that those taking more than 250 IU a day for two years have 41% lower incidence of major heart disease. To take the equivalent of 400 IU in food would require 2 quarts of corn oil or 28 cups of peanuts a day. Vitamin E has a hormonal balance effect that is important to females. Males do not need as much.

Selenium (Antioxidant) – 200 mcg (285 % RDA) in amino acid complex form to enhance absorption. Selenium is a strong antioxidant and the level in our body falls with age. People with decreased levels of selenium are associated with a higher incidence of heart disease, cancer, and arthritis.

Magnesium (Antioxidant) – 500 to 1000 mg (125% to 250% RDA). Less than 25% of Americans meet the low RDA standard. A 2,000 kcal diet is needed if no supplement is taken. This is critical for proper heart function, to normalize arrhythmias, and helps to reduce blood pressure. Requirement is higher if your intake of sugar and fat is high in your diet. The calcium to magnesium ratio should be between 1:1 to 1:2.

Vitamin B9 (Folic acid) – 800 mcg (200% RDA) – a non-toxic nutrient that protects chromosomes from DNA damage and cancer. A Harvard study of 16,000 women and 9,500 men showed that those getting the most folic acid had the lowest incidence of getting pre-cancerous polyps in the colon. Folic acid also helps with depression. No noticeable side effects at up to 10,000 mcg.

Vitamin B12 – 100 to 1,000 mcg (1,666% RDA) – over 24% of people over 60 years old and over 40% of people over 80 years old are deficient due to decreased absorption with age. Deficiency also causes symptoms similar to Alzheimer's disease. A must take for those over 50 years old as a cheap and added insurance. Non-toxic at 1,000 mcg daily for many years or up to 100,000 mcg in a single dose.

Chromium – 200 mcg (166% RDA) in chelated form for better absorption. Very little is contained in food and, as a result, 90% of all Americans are deficient in this trace element, which is critical in order to normalize blood sugar. An Israeli research shows that a daily intake of 200 mcg of chromium improved insulin resistance in Type II Diabetes by up to 50% in weeks.

Zinc – 30 to 50 mg (200% RDA) in chelated form for better absorption. Thirty-three percent of healthy Americans over the age of 50 have zinc deficiency and do not know it. The percentage increases to 90% for those older. You need a daily calorie intake of 2,400 kcal to get just the RDA. Zinc is critical for proper thymus gland and immune system function. Research has shown that daily intake of 30 mg of zinc stimulates the immune system, with dramatic improvements after six months for those with zinc deficiency.

Calcium – 300 to 500 mg (30% to 50% RDA) in the form of calcium carbonate. In addition to keeping our bones healthy, calcium also fights cancer. Calcium carbonate contains 40% calcium, compared to others such as calcium gluconate, which contain 9% elemental calcium. Do not take more than 500 mg at a time for best absorption. Calcium should be balanced with Magnesium at 1:1 or 1:2 ratio.

Citrus Bioflavonoids – 100 mg – potent anti oxidants derived from plants that have metal binding (chelating) properties. Commonly found in grape seed.

Omega 3 Fatty Acid – Not needed if you take 8 oz of fish a week. Otherwise, 2,000 to 3,000 mg of fish oil (each 1,000 mg to contain 360 mg EPA and 240 mg DHA) may be considered. Most people taking fish oil have a tendency to develop a fishy " burp". Over 60 research studies (most using 3,000 mg of fish oil a day) have shown that a variety of ailments from arthritis to heart disease can benefit from fish oil (not cod liver oil, which contains high doses of vitamins A and D, which is toxic); 400 IU of vitamin E should be taken simultaneously to potentiate the effect of fish oil.

Garlic – 500 mg in concentrated form – equivalent to 1,250 mg garlic bulk or half a clove of fresh garlic. Garlic has been used by healers for over 5,000 years. Numerous studies have shown that garlic decreases triglyceride level by decreasing fat absorption. It also supports healthy blood pressure. Garlic's major compounds, allicin, have been found to possess powerful actions that help the body boost its immune power. A natural herb that is non-toxic.

Saw Palmetto – 160 to 320 mg – Saw palmetto is a small palm tree native to the West Indies and the Atlantic coast of North America. The active component helps maintain healthy levels of dihydrotestosterone (DHT) in the prostate, and promote proper excretion of DHT from the prostate. Research has shown that 80% of all males will be afflicted with prostate enlargement, a common condition that is also a leading cause of prostate cancer, by the time a man is 80 years old. One-third of all males above 35 years old already have a predisposition to pre-cancerous prostate lesions, and 50% of all males at age 50 have enlarged prostate. A healthy prostate will also ensure proper urinary and reproductive health. This herb is a non-toxic and risk free prevention of this medical condition.

Digestive Enzyme containing amylase, lactase, protease and cellulase is important to promote gastro-intestinal health.

Avoid **Iron unless You are Anemic.**

IMPORTANT

Vitamin B1 (thiamine) – 100 mg (6666% RDA) –critical for mental function and nerve cell growth. Non-toxic and water soluble.

Vitamin B2 (riboflavin) – 50 mg (2,940% RDA) – required for cell growth and release of energy, formation of red blood cell, and synthesis of antibodies.

Vitamin B3 (niacin) – 190 mg (950% RDA) in the form of niacin and niacinamide – stabilize cell membranes,

Vitamin B5 (panthothenic acid) – 400 mg (4,000% RDA) – a non-toxic nutrient needed to breakdown fat to covert into energy. An anti-stress vitamin.

Vitamin B7 (biotin) – 300 mcg (100% RDA) – essential for protein, fat and carbohydrate metabolism. Helps utilization of other B complex vitamins.

Iodine – 150 mcg (100% RDA) – important to maintain proper thyroid function.

Manganese – 20 mg (1,000% RDA) – trace mineral essential for protein and fat metabolism.

Molybdenum – 50 mcg (66% RDA) – essential trace mineral for nitrogen metabolis.

Potassium – 99 mg – critical for normal cardiac rhythm.

Boron – 2 mg – enhances healthy bone and brain function and alertness.

Vanadium – 25 mcg – essential in the formation of bone and teeth.

L-Lysine – 600 mg – an essential amino acid for proper growth in children and protein synthesis in adults.

Choline – 200 mg – responsible for proper neurotransmitter function, lecithin formation, liver function, and gall bladder regulation.

Inositol – 100 mg – vital for hair growth and prevention of the hardening of arteries.

PABA (Para-Aminobenzoic Acid) – basic constituent of many B complexes and antioxidants. Helps protect against sunburn and skin cancer.

DOSAGE GUIDE

Nutrient		Men RDA	Women RDA	Optimum Daily Allowance	Healthy Adult Safe Range
Beta Carotene	IU	None tested	None tested	10,000 - 30,000	20,000 - 100,000
Biotin	mcg	100 - 200	100 - 200	200 - 500	200 - 800
Boron	mg	None tested	None tested	1 - 3	No known limit
Calcium	mg	800	1,000 -1,500	300 - 500	1,000 - 2,000
Chromium	mg	50-200	50-200	200	100 - 400
Coenzyme Q-10	mg	None tested	None tested	25 - 100	
Copper	mcg	2.0 - 3.0	2.0 - 3.0	2.0 - 3.0	No known limit
Cysteine	mg	None tested	None tested	500 - 1,500	800-300 Take with vitamin B12
Folic Acid	mcg	400	400	400 - 1,000	No known limit
Gultamine	mg	None tested	None tested	500 - 2,000	200
Iodine	mcg	150	150	250	50 - 100
Iron	mg	10	18 (Pre-meno-pausal)	Men:10 mg; Women: (Pre-menopausal:10mg)	400 - 1,000
Lysine	mg	None tested	None tested	500-2,000	400 - 1,000
Magnesium	mg	350	300	400 - 1,000	No known limit
Manganese	mg	None tested	None tested	10	60 - 1,000
Pantothenic acid	mg	4 - 7	4 - 7	10 - 10	
Phosphorus	mg	800	800	1,200	
Postassium	mg	None tested	None tested	Not known, but the recommended number of servings of fruits and vegetables supplies about 3,500 mg per day	15,000
Selenium	mcg	50 - 200	50 - 200	200	100 - 400
Silicon	None tested	None tested	Not known	Not known limit	
Sodium	mg	1,100 - 3,300	1,100 - 3,300	Not known, but most nutitionists recommend 3,000 mg per day or less	

DOSAGE GUIDE

Nutrient		Men RDA	Women RDA	Optimum Daily Allowance	Healthy Adult Safe Range
Sulfur	None tested	None tested	None tested	No known limit	
Taurine	mg	None tested	None tested	500 - 2,000	No known limit
Tyrosine	mg	None tested	None tested	500 - 1,500	No known limit
Vitamin A	IU	3,300	2,664	10,000	5,000 - 20,000
Vitamin B1 (Thiamine)	mg	1.2	1.0	5 - 10	10 - 300
Vitamin B12 (Cobalamin)	mcg	3.0	3.0	500 - 1,000	500 - 2,000
Vitamin B2 (Riboflavin)	mg	1.4	1.2	6 - 15	50 - 250
Vitamin B3 (Niacin)	mg	18	13	25 - 100	Niacin: 10-200 mg: Inositol hexanicotinate: 100-3,000 mg (under a doctor's supervision); Niacinamide: 10-300 mg
Vitamin B6 (Pyridoxine)	mg	2.2	2.0	10 - 20	10-400 mg. Long term use of over 200 mg daily requires a doctor's supervision
Vitamin C	mg	90	75	250 - 3,000	250-10,000 mg depending on individual tolerance
Vitamin D	IU	200	200 - 400	400-15,000 IU, but not normally necessary if you get 20 minutes or more of sun exposure daily	
Vitamin E (natural)	IU	15	15	50 - 800	100-1,200 IU. If you have high blood pressure, 400 IU except under a doctor's supervision
Vitamin K	mcg	70 - 140	70 - 140	same as RDA	50 - 500
Zinc	mg	15	15	15 - 35	15 - 300

REFERENCES

Adlercreutz H: Determination of Urinary Ligans and Phytoestrogens Metabolites, Potential Antiestrogens, and Anticarcinogens, in Urine of Women on Various Diets. *J Steriod Biochem* 25:791, 1986.

Aldercreutz H: Estrogen Metabolism and Excretion in Oriental and Caucasian Women. *J Natl Cancer Inst* 86:1076, 1994.

Adlerercreutz H: Quantitative Determination of Lignans and Isoflavonoids in Plasma of Omnivorous and Vegetarian Women by Isotope Dilution Gas Chromatography-Mass Spectrometry. *Scan J Clin Lab Invest* 215(1):5, 1993.

Agus DB, Vera JC, Golde DW: Stomal Cell Oxidation: A Mechanism by Which Tumors Obtain Vitamin C. *Cancer Research* 59:4555-4558, Sept 1999.

Allison DB, Fontaine KR, Manson JE, Stevens J, Vanltallie TB: Annual Deaths Attributable to Obesity In The United States. *JAMA* 282(16):1530-1538, Oct 1996.

Ambrose J: Thrombosis in Ischemic Heart Disease. *Arch Intern Med* 156:1382, 1996.

American Cancer Society: ACS Guidelines on Diet, Nutrition and Cancer. *Ca Cancer J Clinicians* 41:334-339, 1991.

American Diabetes Association: Nutrition Recommendations and Principles for Individuals with Diabetes Mellitus. 18 May 1994 *(in press)*.

American Dietetic Association: Position of the American Dietetic Association: Vegetarian Diets. *J Am Diet Assoc* 93:1317-1319, 1993.

American Dietetic Association: Position of The American Dietetic Association: Vegetarian Diets," *J Am Diet Assoc* 97:11, November 1997.

American Heart Association: 2000 Heart and Stroke Statistical Update. *(Dallas, Texas: American Heart Association, 1999).*

American Heart Association: 2000 Heart and Stroke Statistical Update: Coronary Heart Disease and Angina Pectoris. *(Dallas, Texas: American Heart Association, 1999).*

American Heart Association: 2000 Heart and Stroke Statistical Update. Risk Factors. *(Dallas, Texas: American Heart Association, 1999).*

American Heart Association: Mediterranean Diet: Does the 'Mediterranean' diet follow AHA dietary guidelines? http://www.Americanheart.org/heart_and_stroke_A_Z_Guide/meddiet.html *(American Heart Association, 2000).*

American Institute for Cancer Research: Dietary Guidelines to Lower Cancer Risk. *(Washington DC, 1990).*

Anderson J: Long-Term Effects of High-Carbohydrate, High-Fiber Diets on Glucose and Lipid Metabolism: a Preliminary Report on Patients With Diabetes. *Diabetes Care* 1:77, 1978.

Anderson JW: Dietary Fibre and Human Health. *Hort Sci* 25:1488-1495, 1990.

Anderson JW, Gustafson NJ, Bryant C.A, et al: Dietary Fiber and Diabetes: A Comprehensive Review and Practical Application. *J AM Diet Assoc* 87:1189-1197, 1987.

Anderson KM, et al: Cholesterol and Mortality: 30 Years of Follow-up from the Framingham Study. *J of the Amer Med Assoc* 257:2176, 1987.

Appel L: A Clinical Trial of the Effects of Dietary Patterns on Blood Pressure. *N Engl Med* 336:1117, 1997.

Appel LJ, Morre T.J, Obarzanek E, Vollmer WM, Svetkey LP, Sacks F.M, Bray GA, Vogt TM, Cutler JA, Windhauser M.M, Lin PH, Karanja N: A Clinical Trial of the Effects of Dietary Patterns on Blood Pressure. (DASH Collaborative Research Group) *N Engl J Med* 336(16): 1117-1124, April 1997.

Armstrong B, Doll R: Environmental Factors and Cancer Incidence and Mortality in Different Countries with Special Reference to Dietary Practices. *Int J Cancer* 15:617-631, 1975.

Arroll B, et al: Does Physical Activity Lower Blood Pressure? A Critical Review Of the Clinical Trials. *J of Clin Epidemiology* 45:419, 1992.

Balch JF, Balch PA: Prescription for Nutritional Healing, 2nd ed. *(Garden City Park: Avery Publishing Group, 1997).*

Beilin LJ, Rouse IL, Armstrong BK, et al: Vegetarian Diet and Blood Pressure Levels: Incidental or Causal Association. *Am J Clin Nutr* 48:806-810, 1988.

Blair SN, Kohl HW 3d, Paffenbarger RS Jr, Clark DG, Cooper KH, Gibbons LW: Physical Fitness and All-cause Mortality: A Prospective Study of Healthy Men and Women. *JAMA* 263:2395-401, 17 November 1989.

Blankenhorn D: Beneficial Effects of Combined Colestipol-Niacin Therapy on Coronary Atherosclerosis and Coronary Venous Bypass Grafts. *JAMA* 257:3233,1987.

Block G, Menkes M: Ascorbic Acid in Cancer Prevention: in Moon TE and M S Micozzi eds. Nutrition and Cancer Prevention: Investigating the role of Micronutrients. *(New York: Marcel and Dekker Inc, 1989).*

Block G, Patterson B, Subar A: Fruit, Vegetables and Cancer Prevention: A Review of the Epidemiological Evidence. *Nutr And Cancer* 18:1-29, 1992.

Bordia A: The Effect of Vitamin C on Blood Lipids, Fibrinolytic Activity and Platelet Adhesiveness in Patients with Coronary Artery Disease. *Atherosclerosis* 35:181, 1980.

Bortz II W.M: Dare to Be 100. *(New York: Simon & Schuster Inc, 1996).*

Boushey CJ, et al: A Quantitative Assessment of Plasma Homocysteine As A Risk Factor For Vascular Disease. *J of Amer Med Assoc* 274:1049, 1995.

Brody J: Natural Chemicals Now Called Major Causes of Disease. *(New York Times, April 26, 1988).*

Brody J: Skipping Breakfast a Poor Way to Start the Day. *Star Tribune* 1:E3(col. 1-4), October, 1998.

Burack OR, et al: The Effects of List-Making On Recall In Young And Elderly Adults. *J of Gerontology, Series B: Psychological and Social Sciences* 51B(4):226, 1996.

Burr ML, Butland BK: Heart Disease in British Vegetarians. *AM J Clin Nutr* 48:830-832, 1988.

Burr ML, Sweetnam PM: Vegetarianism, Dietary Fiber, and Mortality. *AM J Clin Nutr* 36:873-877, 1982.

Burskirk ER, et al: Age And Aerobic Power: The Rate Of Change In Men And Women. *Federation Proceedings* 46:1824, 1987.

Butrum RR, Clifford CK, Lanze E: NCI Dietary Guidelines: Rationale. *AM J Clin Nutr* 48:888-895, 1988.

Butterfield GE, et al: Effect of rhGH and rhIGF-I Treatment On Protein Utilization In Elderly Women. *Amer J of Physiology* E94, 1996.

Campbell WW, et al: Effects of Resistance Training and Dietary Protein Intake on Protein Metabolism In Older Adults. *Amer J of Physiology* 268:1143, 1995.

Carper J: Stop Aging Now! The Ultimate Plan for Staying Young and Reversing the Aging Process. *(New York: HarperCollins Publishers, 1996).*

Carr D: Physical Conditioning Facilitates the Exercise Induced Secretion of Beta-Endorphins and Beta-Lipotropin in Women. *N Engl J Med* 305:560, 1981.

Carroll KK, Kohr HT: Dietary Fat in Relation to Tumorienesis. *Prog Biochem. Pharmoacol* 10:308-353, 1975.

Carroll KK, Braden LM, Bell JA, Kalameghan R: Fat and Cancer. *Cancer* 58:1818-1825, 1986.

Cartmel BL, Loescher J, Villar-Werstler P: Professional and Consumer Concerns about the Environment, Lifestyle and Cancer. *Sem Onol Nurs* 8:20-29, 1992.

Cauley J: Estrogen Replacement Therapy and Mortality among Older Women: The Study of Osteoporotic Fractures. *Arch Intern Med* 157:2181, 1997.

Cauley JA, et al: Estrogen Replacement Therapy and Fractures In Older Women. *Ann Of Intern Med* 122(1):9, 1995.

Cawte J: Parameters of Kava used as a Challenge to Alcohol. *Aust NZ J Psychiatry* 20:70, 1986.

Chopy MC, et al: Vitamin D3 and Calcium to Prevent Hip Fracture in Elderly Women. *N Engl J of Med* 327(23):1637, 1992.

Clark LC, et al: Effects of Selenium Supplementation For Cancer Prevention In Patients with Carinoma Of The Skin. *J of the Amer Med Assoc* 276:1957, 1996.

Clifford C, Kramer B: Diet as Risk and Therapy for Cancer. *Med Clin North Am* 77:725-744. 1993.

Cohen F, Kemeny ME, Kearney KA, Zeagans LS, Neuhaus JM, Conant MA: Persistent Stress as a Predictor of Genital Herpes Recurrence. *Arch Intern Med* 159:2430-2436, November 1999.

Cohen KS: *The Way of Qigong: The Art and Science of Chinese Energy Healing.* (New York: The Ballantine Publishing Group, 1997).

Cohen MR, Doner K: *The Chinese Way to Healing: Many Paths to Wholeness.* (New York: The Berkley Publishing Group, 1996).

Col NF, et al: Patient-Specific Decisions about Hormone Replacement Therapy In Postmenopausal Women. *J of the Amer Med Assoc* 277:1140, 1997.

Colditz G: The Use of Estrogens and Progestins and the Risk of Breast Cancer in Postmenopausal Women. *N Engl J Med* 332:1589, 1995.

Colditz GA, et al: The Use Of Estrogens and Progestins and the Risk Of Breast Cancer In Postmenopausal Women. *N Engl J of Med* 332(24):1589, 1995. *Committee on Diet and Health, Food and Nutrition Board: Commission on Life Sciences, National Research Council. Diet and Health: Implications for Reducing Chronic Disease Risk.* (Washington DC: National Academy Press, 1989).

Compston J: Bone Densitometry in Clinical Practice. *BMJ* 310:1507, 1995.

Corpoas E, et al: Human Growth Hormone and Human Aging. *Endocrine Reviews* 14(1):20, 1993.

Cummings S: Risk Factors for Hip Fracture in White Women. *N Engl J Med* 332:767, 1995.

Dawson-Hughes B, et al: Effect of Calcium And Vitamin D Supplementation Of Bone Density in Men and Women 65 years of Age and Older. *N Engl J of Med* 337:400, 1997.

Delcourt CJ, Cristol, Tessier F, Leger CL, Descomps B, Papoz L, the POLA Study Group: Age-related Macular Degeneration and Antioxidant Status in the POLA Study. *Arch Ophthalmol* 117:1384, October 1999.

Dennerstein L: Progesterone and the Premenstrual Syndrome: a Double Blind Crossover Trial. *BMJ* 290:1617, 1985.

Despres JP, et al: Hyperinsulinemia as an Independent Risk Factor For Ischemic Heart Disease. *N Engl J of Med* 334:952, 1996.

Diaz MN, et al: Antioxidants and Atherosclerotic Heart Disease. *N Engl J of Med* 337:408, 1997.

Dockery DW, Pope III CA, Xu X, Spengler JD, Ware JH, Fay ME, Ferris BG, Speizer E: An Association between Air Pollution and Mortality in Six US Cities. *N Engl J of Med* 329(24):1753-1759, December 1993.

Doll R, Peto R: The Causes of Cancer: Quantitative Estimates of Avoidable Risks of Cancer in the United States Today. *J Nalt Cancer Inst* 66(6):1191-1308, 1981.

Donaldson L: Incidence of Fractures in a Geographically Defined Population. *J Epidemiol Community Health* 44:241, 1990.

Duncan J: Women Walking for Health and Fitness. How Much Is Enough. *JAMA* 266:3295, 1991.

Durazo-Arvizu RA, McGee DL, Cooper RS, Liao Y, Luke A: Mortality and Optimal Body Mass Index in a Sample of the US Population. *AM J Epidemiol* 147(8):739-749, Apr 1998.

Dwyer JT: Health Aspects of Vegetarian Diets. *Am J Clin Nutr* 48:712-738, 1988.

Dwyer JT: Nutritional Consequences of Vegetarianism. *Ann Rev Nutr* 11:61-91, 1991.

Editorial: Development of Molecular Pharmacotherapy. *N Engl J of Med* 342:42-49, 2000.

Editorial: Looking Back on the Millennium in Medicine, Editorial. *N Engl J of Med* 342(1):42-49, January 2000.

Einer-Jensen N: Cimicifuga and Melbrosia Lack Oestrogenic Effects in Mice and Rats. *Maturitas* 25:149, 1996.

Eisenberg DM, Kessler RC, Foster C, Norlock FE, Calikins DR, Delbano TL: Unconventional Medicine in the United States: Prevalence, Cost and Patterns of Use. *N Engl J Med* 328(4):246-252, Jan 1993.

Emmert DH, Kirchner JT: The Role of Vitamin E in the Prevention of Heart Disease. *Arch Fam Med* 8:537-542, November 1999.

Eskinazi D: Homeopathy Re-visited: Is Homeopathy Compatible With Biomedical Observation. *Arch Intern Med* 159:1981-1987, September 1999.

Evans W, Rosenberg IH: *Biomarkers: The 10 Keys to Prolonging Vitality.* (New York: Simon & Schuster Inc, 1992).

Evans WJ: Effects of Exercise On Body Composition And Functional Capacity of The Elderly. *J of Gerontology* 50A:147, 1995.

Fabre C, et al: Effectiveness of Individualized Aerobic Training At The Ventilatory Threshold In The Elderly. *J of Perontology: Biological Sciences* 52A(5):B260, 1997.

Fine JT, Colditz GA, Coakly EH, Moseley G, Manson JE, Willett WC, Kawachi I: A Prospective Study of Weight Change and Health-Related Quality of Life in Women. *JAMA* 282(22):2136-2138, December 1999.

Fink JM: *Third Opinion: An International Directory to Alternative Therapy Centers for the Treatment and Prevention of Cancer & Other Degenerative Diseases, 2nd ed.* (Garden City Park: Avery Publishing Group, 1997).

Fischer ID, Brown DR, Blanton CJ, Casper ML, Croft JB, Brownson RC: Physical Activity Patterns of Chippewa and Menominee Indians: The Inter-Tribal Heart Project. *Amer J of Prev Med* 17(3):189-197, October 1999.

Fraser GE: Determinants of Ischemic Heart Disease in the Seventh Day Adventists: A Review. *AM J Clin Nutr* 48:833-836, 1988.

Freeland-Graves J: Mineral Adequacy of Vegetarian Diets. *AM J Clin Nutr* 48:859-62, 1988.

Fried LP, Borhani NO, Enright P, Furberg CD, Gardin JM, Kronmal RA, Kuller LH, Manolio TA, Mittelmark MB, Newman A: The Cardiovascular Health Study: Design and Rationale. *Ann Epidemiol* 1(3):263-276, February 1991.

Gallagher D, Visser M, Sepulveda D, Pierson RN, Harris T, Heymsfield SB: How useful is Body Mass Index for Comparison of Body Fatness Across Age, Sex and Ethnic Groups?" *Am J Epidemiol* 143(3):228-39, February 1996.

Galland L: Immune Power for Kids. http://healthy.net/library/coloumns/galland/archive/16immunekids.asp *(Healthy.Net, 2000).*

Garfinkel L: Overweight and Cancer. *Ann Intern Med* 103(6):1034-1036(Part 2), December 1985.

Garrison RJ, Castelli WP: Weight and Thirty-Year Mortality of Men in the Framingham Study. 103(6):1006-9(Pt 2), December 1985.

Gillman MW, Cupples A, Millen BE, et al: Inverse Association of Dietary Fat with Development of Ischemic Stroke in Men. *JAMA* 278:2145-50, 1997.

Gisolfi C, Maughan R, Schiller L, Heitlinger L, Rhoads JM, Wapnir RA: Intestinal Fluid Absorption in Exercise and Disease. *Sports Science Exchange Roundtable* 4(1), 1993.

Glaser R, Rabin B, Chesney M, Cohen S, Natelson B: Reductions in Motor Vehicle Related Injuries and Deaths. *JAMA* 282(23):2210-2213, December 1999.

Glass TA, Leon Mde, Marottoli A: Population Based Study of Social and Productive Activities as Predictors of Survival Among Elderly Americans. *British Med Journal* 319:478-483, August 1999.

Gottleib S: US Relaxes its Guidelines on Herbal Supplements. *British Med J* 320(207), January 2000.

Graham TE, Spriet LL: Caffeine and Exercise Performance. *Sports Science Exchange* 9(1), 1996.

Graham, et al: Selenium And Cancer Prevention: Promising Results Indicate Further Trials Required (editorial). *J of Amer Med Assoc 276:24*, December 1996.

Grodstein F, et al: Postmenopausal Hormone Therapy and mortality. *N Engl J of Med* 336:1769,1997.

Grundy S.M, Balady GJ, Criqui MH, Fletcher G, Greenland P, Hiratzka LF, Housten-Miller LM, Kris-Etherton P, Krumholz HM, LaRosa J, Ockene IS, Pearson TA, Reed J, Washington R, Smith S: Primary Prevention of Coronary Heart Disease: Guidance

From Framingham. (A Statement for Healthcare Professionals From the AHA Task Force on Risk Reduction). *Circulation* 97:1876-1887, 1998.

Gustafson N: *Vegetarian Nutrition.* (San Marcos, CA: Nutrition Dimension, 1994).

Haddad EH: Development of a Vegetarian Food Guide. *Amer J of Clin Nutr* 59:1248s-1254s, 1994.

Hahn RA, Teutsch SM, Rothenberg RM, Marks JS: Excess Deaths from Nine Chronic Diseases in the United States. *JAMA*, 264(20):2654-2659, November 1990.

Haines C: Dietary Calcium Intake in Postmenopausal Chinese Women. *Eur J Clin Nutr* 48:591, 1994.

Hamalainen E: Diet and Serum Sex Hormones in Healthy Men. *J Steriod Biochem* 20:459, 1984.

Hamm M, Hauswirtschalf FEU, Hamburg F: Ensuring a Balanced Vegetarian Diet. *Sports Science Update* 1(2), November 1995.

Harris MI, Flegal KM, Cowie CC, Eberhardt MS, Goldstein DE, Little RR, Wiedmeyer HM, Byrd-Holt DD: Prevalence of Diabetes, Impaired Fasting Glucose, and Impaired Glucose Tolerance in the U.S. Adults, The Third National Health and Nutrition Examination Survey, 1988-1994. *Diabetes Care* 21(4):518-524, April 1998.

Hart CL, Hole DJ, Smith GD: Risk Factors and 20-Year Stroke Mortality in Men and Women in Renfrew/Paisley Study in Scotland. *Stroke* 30(10):1999-2007, October 1999.

Hartz AJ, Kuhn EM, Bentler SE, Levine PH, London R: Prognostic Factors for Persons With Idiopathic Chronic Fatigue. *Arch Fam Med* 8:495-501, November 1999.

Haskell W: Effects of Intensive Multiple Risk Factor Reduction on Coronary Atherosclerosis and Clinical Cardiac Events in Men and Women with Coronary Artery Disease: the Stanford Coronary Risk Intervention Project (SCRIP). *Circulation* 89:975, 1994.

Hegsted M: Urinary Calcium and Calcium Balance in Young Men as Affected by Level of Protein and Phosphorus Intake. *J Nutr* 111:553, 1981.

Health Study: Design and Rationale. *Ann Epidemiol* 1(3):263-276, February 1991.

Hermanson B, et al: Beneficial Six Year Outcome of Smoking Cessation in Older Men And Women with Coronary Artery Disease. *N Engl J Med* 319:1365, 1988.

Higgins MW, et al: Smoking And Lung Function In Elderly Men And Women. *J of the Amer Med Assoc* 269:2741, 1993.

Hirayama T: Epidemiology of Breast Cancer With Special Reference to the Role of Diet. *Prev Med* 7:173-195, 1978.

Ho S: Determinants of Bone Mass in the Chinese Old-Old Population. *Osteoporos Int* 5:161, 1995.

Hochberg MC, Lethbridge-Cejku M, Scott Jr WW, Reichle R, Plato CC, Tobin JD: The Association of Body Weight, Body Fatness and Body Fat Distribution with Osteoarthritis of the Knee: Data from the Baltimore Longitudinal Study of Aging. *J Rheumatol* 22(3):488-493, March 1995.

Hoes A: Diuretics, Beta-Blockers, and the Risk for the Sudden Cardiac Death in Hypertensive Patients. *Ann Intern Med* 123:481, 1995.

Hoffman C: Persons with Chronic Conditions: Their Prevalence and Costs. *JAMA* 276:1473, 1996.

Holloszy J O, et al: Effects Of Exercise On Glucose Tolerance And Insulin Resistance. *Acta Medica Scandinavia* 711(1):55, 1986.

Holloway L: Effects of Recombinant Human Growth Hormone On Metabolic Indices, Body Composition, And Bone Turnover In Healthy Elderly Women. *J of Clin Endrocrinology Metabolism* 79:470.

Hopkins G J, Carroll KK: Role of Diet in Cancer prevention. *J Environ Pathol Toxicol Oncol* 5:279-298, 1985.

Hopper J: The Bone Density of Female Twins Discordant for Tobacco Use. *N Engl J Med* 330:387, 1994.

Howard J.M, Azen C, Jacobsen DW, Green R, Carmel R: Dietary Intake of Cobalamin in Elderly People who have Abnormal Serum Cobalamin, Methylmalonic Acid and Homocysteine Levels. 52(8):582-587, August 1998.

Howe GR, Friedenreich CM, Jain M, Miller AB: A Cohort Study of Fat Intake and Risk of Breast Cancer. *J Natl Cancer Inst* 83:336-340, 1991.

Hu J: Dietary Intakes and Urinary Excretion of Calcium and Acids: a Cross-Sectional Study of Women in China. *Am J Clin Nutr* 58:398, 1993.

Hunt C, Chakravorty NK, Annan G: The Clinical and Biochemical Effects of Vitamin C Supplementation in Short-Stay Hospitalized Geriatric Patients. *Int J Vitam Nutr Res* 54(1):65-74, 1984.

Ip C: Review of the effects of Trans Fatty Acids, Oleic Acid, n-3 Polyunsaturated Fatty Acids, and Conjugated Linoleic Acid on Mammary Carcinogenesis in Animals. *AM J Clin Nutr* 66: 1523S, 1997.

Itoh R: Dietary Protein Intake and Urinary Excretion of Calcium: a Cross-Sectional Study in Healthy Japanese Population. *AM J Clin Nutr* 67:438, 1998.

Itoh R: Sodium Excretion in Relation to Calcium and Hydroxyproline Excretion in Japanese Population. *AM J Clin Nutr* 63:735, 1996.

Jacques PF, Selhub J, Bostom AG, Wilson PWF, Rosenberg DIH: The Effect of Folic Acid Fortification on Plasma Folate and Total Homocysteine Concentrations. *The New England J of Med* 340(19):1449-1454, May 1999.

Jain A: Can Garlic Reduce the Levels of Serum Lipids? A Controlled Clinical Study. *Am J Med* 94:632, 1993.

Jakicic JM, Winters C, Lang W, Wing RR: Effects of intermittent Exercise and Use of Home Exercise Equipment on Adherence, Weight Loss, and Fitness in Overweight Women. *JAMA* 282(16):1554-1560, October 1999.

Jenkins D: Wholemeal versus Wholegrain Breads: Proportion of Whole or Cracked Grain and the Glycaemic Response. *BMJ* 297:958, 1988.

Jensen OM, MacLennon R, Wahrendorf J: Diet, Bowel function, Fecal characteristics and Large Bowel Cancer in Denmark and Finland. *Nutr Cancer* 4:5-19, 1982.

Jeste DV, Alexpoulos GS, Bartels SJ, Cummings JL, Gallo JJ, Gottleib GL, Halpain MC, **Palmer BW, Patterson TL, Reynolds CF, Lebowitz DBD:** Consensus Statement on the Upcoming Crisis in Geriatric Mental Health. Research Agenda For The Next 2 Decades. *Arch. Gen. Psychiatry* 56:848-853, September 1999.

Jha P, et al: The Antioxidant Vitamins and Cardiovascular Disease. *Ann Of Intern Med* 123:860, 1995.

Johnston CS: Recommendations for Vitamin C Intake. *JAMA* 282(22), December 1999.

Joint Nutrition Monitoring Evaluation Committee Report, Nutrition Monitoring in the United States: an Update Report on Nutrition Monitoring: Executive Summary. *Nutr Today* 25(1):33-42, 1990.

Kahn RH, Philips RL, Snowdon DA, et al: Association between Reported Diet and all Cause Mortality: Twenty -one Year Follow Up on 27, 530 Adult Seventh-Day Adventists. *Am J Epidemiol* 119:775-787, 1984.

Kannus P: Effect of Starting Age of Physical Activity on Bone Mass in the Dominant Arm of Tennis and Squash Players. *Ann Intern Med* 123:27, 1995.

Kant AK, Schatzkin A, Graubard BI, Schairer C: A Prospective Study of Diet Quality and Mortality in Women. *JAMA* 283(16):2109-2115, April 2000.

Kasch FW, Boyer JL, Schmidt PK, Wells RH, Wallace JP, Verity LS, Guy H, Schneider D: Aging of the Cardiovascular System During 33 Years of Aerobic Exercise. *Age and Aging* 28:531-536, 1999.

Katzel LI, et al: Effects Of Weight Loss Vs. Aerobic Exercise Training On Risk Factors For Coronary Disease In Healthy, Obese, Middle-aged, and Older Men. *J of the Amer Med Assoc* 274:1915, 1995.

Kelley G, et al: Antihypertensive Effects Of Aerobic Exercise: A Brief Meta-Analytic Review Of Randomized Controlled Trials. *Amer J of Hyertension* 7:115, 1994.

Key TJ, Fraser GE, Thorogood M, et al: Mortality in Vegetarians and Non-Vegetarians: A Collaborative Analysis of 8300 Deaths Among 76,000 Men and Women in Five Prospective Studies. *Public Health Nutrition* 1:33-43, 1988.

Kiehm T: Beneficial Effects of a High Carbohydrate, High Fiber Diet on Hyperglycemia in Diabetic Men. *AM J Clin Nutr* 29:895, 1976.

Kineman RD, Kamegai J, Frohman LA: Growth Hormone (hGH)-Releasing Hormone (GHRH) and the GH Secretagogue (GHS), L692,585, Differentially Modulate Rat Pituitary GHS Receptor and GHRH Receptor Messenger Ribonucleic Acid Levels. *Endocrinology* 140(8):3581-86, August 1999.

Kinney AY, Choi YA, DeVellis B, Kobetz E, Millikan RC, Sandler RS: Interest in Genetic Testing Among First Degree Relatives of Colorectal Cancer Patients. *American Journal of Preventive Medicine* 18(3):249-252, April 2000.

Kita Joe: Live to 90 (and die having sex): includes related articles on being smart about health: a 65-year old personal trainer. *Men's Health* 13:132-137, June 1998.

Klatz R, Kahn C: *Grow Young with hGH.* (New York: Harper Collins Publishers, 1997).

Klatz R, Goldman R: *Stopping the Clock.* (New Canaan: Keats Publishing Inc., 1996).

Kleiner SM: The Role of Meat in an Athlete's Diet.: Its Effect on Key Macro-And Micronutrients. *Sports Science Exchange* 8(5), 1995.

Kleinjnen J: Gingko Biloba. *Lancet* 340:1136, 1992.

Knuiman J: HDL-Cholesterol in Men From Thirteen Countries (letter). *Lancet* 2:367, 1981.

Knutsen SF: Lifestyle and the Use of Health Services. *AM J Clin Nutr* 59:1171-1175s, 1994.

Koplan JP, Dietz WH: Caloric Imbalance and Public Health Policy. *JAMA* 282(16):1579-1581, October 1999.

Kramer AM: Health Care for the Elderly Persons – Myths and Realities. *N Engl J of Med* 332(15):1027-1029, April 1995.

Kromhout D, Bosschieter EB, Lezenne-Coulander D: Dietary Fibre and 10 year Mortality from Coronary Heart disease, Cancer, and all Causes. *Lancet* 2:518-522, 1982.

Kuller LH, Shemanski L, Psaty BM, Borhani NO, Gardin J, Hann MN, O'Leary DH, Savage PJ, Tell GS, Tracy R: Subclinical Disease as an Independent Risk Factor for Cardiovascular Disease. *Circulation* 92:720-726, 1995.

Kushi LH, Lenart EB, Willett WC: Health Implications of Mediterranean Diets in the Light of Contemporary Knowledge: Meat, Wine, Fats and Oils. *AM J Clin Nutr* 61:1416-1427s, 1995.

Kushi LH, et al: Dietary Antioxidant vitamins and Death from Coronary Heart Disease In Postmenopausal Women. *N Engl J of Med* 334:1156, 1996.

Kushi LH, Sellers TA, Potter JD, Nelson CL, Munger R G, Kaye S A, Folsom A R: Dietary Fat and Post Menopausal Breast Cancer. *J Natl Cancer Inst* 84:1092-1099, 1992.

Landis S: Cancer Statistics, 1998. *CA Cancer J Clin* 48:6, 1998.

Landon JF, Heck KE, Brett KM: Hormone Replacement Therapy And Breast Cancer Risk In A Nationally Representative Cohort. *Amer J of Prev Med* 17(3):176-180, October 1999.

Lange S: Be Cautious about Using HRT for Women Without Symptoms of Oestrogen Deficiency (letter). *BMJ* 314:1415, 1997.

Lean M: Impairment of Health and Quality of Life in People with Large Waist Circumference. *Lancet* 351:853, 1998.

LeBars P: A Placebo-Controlled, Double-Blind, Randomized Trial of an Extract of Gingko Biloba for Dementia. *JAMA* 278:1327, 1997.

Lee CD, Blair SN, Jackson AS: Cardiorespiratory Fitness, Body Composition, and All-cause and Cardiovascular Disease Mortality in men. *AM J Clin Nutr* 69(3):373-380, March 1999.

Leggatt V, Mackay J, Yates JRW: Evaluation of Questionnaire on Cancer Family History in the Identifying Patients at Increased Genetic Risk in the General Practice. *BMJ* 319(7212):757-758, September 1999.

Lehmann M, Gottfries CG, Regland B: Identification of Cognitive Impairment in the Elderly: Homocysteine is an Early Marker. *Dement Geriatr Cogn Disord* 10(1): 12-20, Jan-Feb 1999.

Libov C: *Beat Your Risk Factors: A Woman's Guide to Reducing Her Risk for Cancer, Heart Disease, Stroke, Diabetes, and Osteoporosis.* (New York: Plume, Penguin Group, 1999).

Lindsted K, Tonstad S, Kuzma JW: Body Mass Index and Patterns of Mortality among Seventh Day Adventist Men. *Int J Obes* 15(6):397-406, June 1991.

Lonn EM, Yusuf S: Emerging Approaches in Preventing Cardiovascular Disease. *Brit Med J* 318:1337-1341, May 1999.

Lowe LP, Greenland P, Ruth KJ, Dyer AR, Stamler R, Stamler J: Impact of Major Cardiovascular Disease Risk Factors, Particularly in Combination, on 22-year Mortality in Women and Men. *Arch Intern Med* 158(18):2007-14, October 1998.

Magaziner A: *The Complete Idiot's Guide to Living Longer & Healthier.* (New York: Simon & Schuster Macmillan Publishing, 1999).

Malhotra SL: Dietary Factors in the Study of Colon Cancer from Cancer Registry, with Special Reference to The Role of Saliva, Milk, and Fermented Milk Products and Vegetable Fibre. *Medical Hypotheses* 3:122-126, 1977.

Mangle R: A Review of Recent Scientific Papers Related to Vegetarianism. *Vegetarian Journal* 17(1), January 1998.

Mansell P: Garlic: Effects on Serum Lipids, Blood Pressure, Coagulation, Platelet Aggregation, and Vasodilatation. *BMJ* 303:379, 1991.

Manson J: Body Weight and Mortality among Women. *N Engl J of Med* 333:677, 1995.

Manson JE, Stampfer MJ, Hennekens CH, Willett WC: Body Weight and Longevity. A Reassessment. *JAMA* 257(3):353-358, Jan 1987.

Manton K G: Longevity in the United States: age and sex specific evidence on life span limits from mortality patterns 1960-1990. *Journal of Gerontology: Biological Sciences* 51A:362, 1996.

Manton K G, Stallard E: Changes In Health, Mortality, And Disability And their Impact On Long term Care Needs. *J of Aging and Social Policy* 7(3/4):25, 1996.

Margetts BM, Beilin LJ, Armstrong BK, et al: Vegetarian Diet in Mild Hypertension: Effects of Fat and Fiber. *AM J Clin Nutr* 48:801-805, 1988.

Martin GM: *Genetics Of Human Disease, Longevity And Aging: In Andres, REL Bierman, WR Hazzard: Principles of Geriatic Medicine.* (New York: McGraw-Hill, 1985).

Martin-Moreno, Boyle JM P, Gorgojo L, Willett WC, Gonzalez J, Villar F, Maisonneuv P: Alcoholic Beverage Consumption and Risk of Breast Cancer in Spain. *Cancer Causes Control* 4:345-353, 1993.

McCaddon A, Davies G, Hudson P, Tandy S, Cattell H: Total Serum Homocysteine in Senile Dementia of Alzheimer Type. *Int J Geriatr Psychiatry* 13(4):235-9, April 1998.

McDougall J: Rapid Reduction of Serum Cholesterol and Blood Pressure by a Twelve-Day, very Low Fat, Strictly Vegetarian Diet. *J Am Coll Nutr* 14:491, 1995.

McDougall JA: *The McDougall Program for Women.* (New York: Plume, Penguin Group, 2000).

McKirnan M: Clinical Significance of Coronary Vascular Adaptions to Exercise in Training. *Med Sci Sports Exerc* 26:1262, 1994.

Mediterranean *Diet for Cancer Prevention.* http://online.com/ch1/in-depth/item/item, 4769_1_1.asp (Massachusetts Medical Society, August 1996).

Mersey D: *Health Benefits of Aerobic Exercise. Postgrad Med 90: Food as Medicine.* (New York: Simon & Schuster Inc, 1994).

Mindell E: Earl Mindell's Supplement 103, 1991.

Mills PK, Beeson WL, Phillips RL, Fraser GE: Cancer Incidence Among California Seventh-day Adventists. *AM J Clin Nutr* 59:1136s-1142s, 1994.

Mindell E: Earl Mindell's Bible. *(New York: Simon & Schuster Inc, 1998).*

Montague CT, Prins JB, Sanders L, Digby JE, Rahilly DSO': Depot- and Sex-Specific Differences in Human Leptin mRNA Expression: Implications for the Control of Regional Fat Distribution. *Diabetes* 46(3):342-347, March 1997.

Morley JE, et al: Geriatric Nutrition: A Comprehensive Review Vol. 45. *(New York: Raven Press, 1990).*

Murphy JE, et al: The Relationship of school breakfast to psychosocial and academic functioning. *Archives of pediatrics and adolescent Medicine* 152(9):899-907, September 1998.

Murray M, Pizzorno J: *Encyclopedia of Natural Medicine, 2nd ed.* (Rocklin: Prima Publishing, 1998).

Mutch PB: Food Guides for the Vegetarian. *Amer J of Clin Nutr* 48:913-919, 1988.

National Academy of Sciences: Fluid Replacement and Heat Stress Committee on Military Nutrition Research Food and Nutrition Board, pp 254, 1994.

National Cholesterol Education Program, Second Report of the Expert Panel on Detention, Evaluation, and Treatment of High Blood Cholesterol in adults. *NIH Publication No.* 93-3095. National Heart Lung and Blood Institute, 1993.

National Institute On Aging, Alzheimer's Disease And Related Dementias: Biomedical Update. (Washington, D.C : Department of Health and Human Services, August 1995).

National Research Council. Committee on Diet, Nutrition, and Cancer, Assembly of Life Sciences, Diet Nutrition and Cancer. (Washington D. C.: National Academy Press, 1982).

National Research Council. Committee on Diet and Health, Food and Nutrition Board, Commission of Life Sciences, Diet and Health: Implications for Reducing Chronic Disease risk (Washington DC: National Academy Press, 1989).

National Task Force on the Prevention and Treatment of Obesity: Overweight, Obesity, and Health Risk. *Arch Intern Med* 160(7):898-904, April 2000.

Naurath H, et al: Effects of Vitamin B12, Folate, And Vitamin B6 Supplements In Elderly People With Normal Serum Vitamin Levels. *Lancet* 346:85, 1995.

Newell SA, Girgis A, Sanson-Fisher RW, Savolainen NJ: The Accuracy of Self Reported Health Behaviours and Risk Factors Relating to Cancer and Cardiovascular Disease in the **General Population:** A Critical Review. *Ameri J of Prev Med* 17(3):211-229, October 1999.

Nikkila E: Prevention of Progression of Coronary Atherosclerosis by Treatment of Hyerlipidaemia: a Seven-Year Prospective Angiographic Study. *Br Med J* 289:220, 1984.

Null G: *Gary Null's Ultimate Anti-Aging Program.* (New York: Kensington Publishing Corp, 1999)

Ornish D: Can Lifestyle Changes Reverse Coronary Heart Disease. *Lancet* 336:129, 1990.

Paffenbarger RS Jr, Hyde R T, Wing AL, Lee IM, Jung DL, Kampert JB: The association of Changes in the Physical Activity Level and Other Lifestyle Characteristics with Mortality Among Men. *N Engl J of Med* 328(8):538-545, February 1993.

Palmer R: Is Breakfast the Most Important Meal of the Day? *Arch Pediatr Adolesc Med* 152:899-907, 1998.

Papadakis MA, et al: Growth Hormone Replacement In Healthy Older Men Improves Body Composition But Not Functional Ability. *Annals of Intern Med* 124:708, 1996.

Parkin DM, Muir CS, Whelan SL, Gao YT, Ferlay J, Powell J: *Cancer Incidence in Five Continents, vol. 6.* (France: Leon, International Agency on Research for Cancer, 1992).

Pesmen C: *How a Man Ages?* (New York: Esquire Press, 1984).

Peterson G: Genistein Inhibition of the Growth of Human Cancer cells: Independence from Estrogens and Multi-Drug Resistance Gene. *Biochem Biophys Res Com* 179:661, 1991.

Petrie K, et al: Effect of Melatonin On Jet Lag After Long Haul Flights. *British Med J* 28:705, 1989.

Phillips B: *Body for Life.* (New York: HarperCollins Publishers, 1999).

Phillips RL, Snowdon DA: Association of Meat and Coffee Use with Cancers of the Large Bowel, Breast, and Prostate among Seventh-Day Adventists: Preliminary Results. *Cancer Res* 45:5403-8, 1983.

Porter DJ, Raymond LW, Anastasio G D: Chromium: Friend or Foe? *Arch Fam Med* 8:386-390, Sep/Oct 1999.

Prince RL: Diet And The Prevention of Osteoporotic Fractures. *N Engl J of Med* 337:701, 1997.

Prince RL, et al: Prevention of Postmenopausal Osteoporosis. A Comparative Study Of Exercise, Calcium Supplementation, and Hormone Replacement Therapy. *N Engl J of Med* 325(17):1189, 1991.

Psaty B: The Risk of Myocardial Infarction with Antihypertensive Drug Therapies. *JAMA* 274:620, 1995.

Qureshi A: Lowering of Serum Cholesterol in the Hypercholestrolemic Humans by Tocotrienols(palmvitee). *AM J Clin Nutr* 53:1021s, 1991.

Raglin J: Exercise and Mental Health. Beneficial and Detrimental Effects. *Sports Med* 9:323, 1990.

Reaven G, Strom TK, Fox Syndrome X B: *Overcoming the Silent Killer that Can Give You a Heart Attack.* (New York: Simon & Schuster Inc., 2000).

Reichel W: *Care Of Elderly: Clinical Aspects of Aging* (4th ed, pp 229, Baltimore: Williams and Wilkins, 1995).

Relman AS, Weil A: Is Integrative Medicine the Medicine of the Future?: A Debate Between Arnold S Relman MD and Andrew Weil MD. *Arch Intern Med* 159:2122-2126, October 1999.

Report of Advisory Committee on the dietary guidelines for Americans 1990. *Nutr Today* 25(4):44-45, 1991.

Rich-Edwards JW, Manson JE, Stampfer MJ, Colditz GA, Willett WC, Rosner B, Speizer FE, Henekkens CH: Height and the Risk of Cardiovascular Disease in Women. *Am J Epidemiol* 142(9):909-917, November 1995.

Richman J: *I'm Too Young to Get Old.*

Rimm E B, et al: Vitamin E Consumption and The Risk of Coronary Heart Disease In Men. *N Engl J of Med* 328(20):1450, 1993.

Ritchie K, Gilham C, Ledesert B, Touchon J, Kotzki PO: Depressive Illness, Depressive Symptomatology and Regional Cerebral Blood Flow in Elderly People with Sub-Clinical Cognitive Impairment. *Age and Aging* 28:385-391, 1999.

Roberts W: Atherosclerotic Risk Factors – Are There Ten or Are There only One. *Am J Cardiol* 64:552, 1989.

Rockhill B, Willett WC, Hunter DJ, Manson JE, Hankinson SE, Colditz GA: A Prospective Study of Recreational Physical Activity and Breast Cancer Risk. *Arch Intern Med* 159:2290-2296, October 1999.

Rogers MA, et al: Changes In Skeletal Muscle With Aging: Effects Of Exercise Training. *Exercise and Sport Science Reviews* 21:65, 1993.

Rohan TE, Baina CJ: Diet in the Etiology of Breast Cancer. *Epidemiol Rev* 9:120-141, 1987.

Roizen MF: Real Age: *Are You as Young as You Can Be?* (New York: HarperCollins Publishers, 1999).

Rose W: The Requirements of Adult Man, XVI. The Role of the Nitrogen Intake. *J Biol Chem* 217:997, 1955.

Ross P: Osteoporosis. Frequency, Consequences, and Risk Factors. *Arch Intern Med* 156:1399, 1996.

Ross P: Pain and Disability Associated with New Vertebral Fractures and other Spine Conditions. *J Clin Epidemiol* 47:231, 1994.

Ross P: Pre-existing Fractures and Bone Mass Predict Vertebral Fracture Incidence in Women. *Ann Intern Med* 114:919, 1991.

Rowe JW: *Toward Successful Aging: Limitation Of The Morbidity Associated With Normal Aging. Principles of Geriatic Med And Gerontology, 2nd ed. (New York: McGraw-Hill, 1990),* pp138.

Rowe JW, Kahn RL: *Successful Aging.* (New York: Dell Publishing, 1999).

Rudman D, et al: Effects of Human Growth Hormone In Men Over 60 Years Old. *N Engl J of Med* 323:1, 1990.

Ryback D: *Look Ten Years Younger, Live Ten Years Longer: A Man's Guide.* (New York: BBS Publishing Corporation, 1995).

Sacks FM, Kass EH: Low Blood Pressure in Vegetarians: Effects of Specific Foods and Nutrients. *AM J Clin Nutr* 48:739-48, 1988.

Sahota O, Masud T: Osteoporosis: Fact, Fiction, Fallacy and the Future. *Age and Aging* 28:425-428, 1999.

Salenius J: Long Term Effects of Guar Gum on Lipid Metabolism after Carotid Endarterectomy. *BMJ* 310:95, 1995.

Sandler RS, Lyles CM, Peipins LA, McAuliffe CA, Woosley JT, Kupper LL: Diet and Risk of Colorectal Adenomas: Macronutrients, Cholesterol and Fiber. *J Natl Cancer Inst* 85: 884-891, 1993.

Schaefer EJ, et al: Lipoprotein (a) Levels And Risk of Coronary Heart Disease in Men. *J of the Amer Med Assoc* 271:999, 1994.

Schreiber G: Weight Modification Efforts by Black and White Pre-adolescent Girls: National Heart, Lung, and Blood Institute Growth and Health Study. *Pediatrics* 63, 1996.

Seeman T, et al: Predicting Changes in Physical Functioning in a High Functioning Elderly Cohort: MacArthur Studies of Successful Aging. *J of Gerontology* 49:M97, 1994.

Seitz HK, Simanowski UA, Osswald BR: Epidemiology and Pathophysiology of Ethanol-associated Gastrointestinal Cancer. *Pharmacogenetics* 2:278-287, 1992.

Selhub J: Association between Plasma Homocysteine Concentrations and Extra-cranial Carotid-artery stenosis. *N Engl J Med* 332:286, 1995.

Selhub J: Vitamin Status and Intake as Primary Determinants of Homocysteinemia in an Elderly Population. *JAMA* 270:2693, 1993.

Sherwin R, Price TR: Fat Chance: Diet and Ishemic Stroke. *JAMA* 278:2185-2186, 1997.

Shultz TD, Howie BJ: In Vitro Binding of Steriod Hormones by Natural and Purified Fibers. *Nutr Cancer* 8:141-147, 1986.

Sinatra ST: *Heartbreak and Heart Disease, A Mind/Body Prescription for Healing the Heart.* (New Canaan: Keats Publishing Inc., 1996).

Sinatra ST: *Optimum Health, A Natural Lifesaving Prescription for Your Body and Mind.* (New York: Bantam Doubleday Dell Publishing Group, Inc., 1997).